NUTRITION AND DIET RESEARCH PROGRESS

CHILD NUTRITION PROGRAMS

BACKGROUND AND CURRENT ISSUES

NUTRITION AND DIET RESEARCH PROGRESS

Additional books and e-books in this series can be found on Nova's website under the Series tab.

NUTRITION AND DIET RESEARCH PROGRESS

CHILD NUTRITION PROGRAMS

BACKGROUND AND CURRENT ISSUES

DANIEL D. COLEMAN
EDITOR

nova
New York

NOTICE TO THE READER

Library of Congress Cataloging-in-Publication Data

ISBN: 978-1-53615-764-2

Published by Nova Science Publishers, Inc. † New York

CONTENTS

Preface		**vii**
Chapter 1	Child Nutrition Programs: Current Issues *Kara Clifford Billings*	**1**
Chapter 2	An Introduction to Child Nutrition Reauthorization *Kara Clifford Billings and* *Randy Alison Aussenberg*	**33**
Chapter 3	School Meals Programs and Other USDA Child Nutrition Programs: A Primer (Updated) *Kara Clifford Billings and* *Randy Alison Aussenberg*	**39**
Chapter 4	Summer Meals: Actions Needed to Improve Participation Estimates and Address Program Challenges *United States Government Accountability Office*	**89**
Chapter 5	Summer Meals: Improvements Needed to Address Participation Estimates and Program Challenges *Kathryn A. Larin*	**151**

Chapter 6	A Primer on WIC: The Special Supplemental Nutrition Program for Women, Infants, and Children (Updated) *Randy Alison Aussenberg*	**165**
Chapter 7	WIC: USDA's Review of Vegetables Available under the Program Followed Leading Research Practices *United States Government Accountability Office*	**203**
Chapter 8	Supplemental Nutrition Assistance Program: Observations on Employment and Training Programs and Efforts to Address Program Integrity Issues *Kathryn Larin*	**217**
Index		**249**
Related Nova Publications		**257**

PREFACE

The term child nutrition programs refers to several U.S. Department of Agriculture Food and Nutrition Service (USDA-FNS) programs that provide food for children in institutional settings. These include the school meals programs—the National School Lunch Program and School Breakfast Program—as well as the Child and Adult Care Food Program, Summer Food Service Program, Special Milk Program, and Fresh Fruit and Vegetable Program. Chapter 1 provides an overview of these and other current issues in the child nutrition programs.

The child nutrition programs and the Special Supplemental Nutrition Program for Women, Infants, and Children (WIC) were last reauthorized in 2010 as reported in chapter 2. Chapter 3 describes how each program operates under current law, focusing on eligibility rules, participation, and funding. This introductory section describes some of the background and principles that generally apply to all of the programs; subsequent sections go into further detail on the workings of each. Chapter 4 examines what is known about SFSP participation, other programs that help feed low-income children over the summer, and challenges, if any, in providing summer meals to children and the extent to which USDA provides assistance to address these challenges.

Chapter 5 is the statement of Kathryn A. Larin on improvements needed in the summer meals program. Chapter 6 provides an overview of the WIC program, including administration, funding, eligibility, benefits, benefits redemption, and cost containment policies. Chapter 7 assesses the extent to which leading research practices were followed in USDA's most recent review of vegetables available under WIC. Chapter 8 discusses SNAP E&T programs, including program participants, design, and USDA oversight, and USDA's efforts to address SNAP program integrity, including improper payments, as well as recipient and retailer fraud.

Chapter 1 - The term *child nutrition programs* refers to several U.S. Department of Agriculture Food and Nutrition Service (USDA-FNS) programs that provide food for children in institutional settings. These include the school meals programs—the National School Lunch Program and School Breakfast Program—as well as the Child and Adult Care Food Program, Summer Food Service Program, Special Milk Program, and Fresh Fruit and Vegetable Program. The most recent child nutrition reauthorization, the Healthy, Hunger-Free Kids Act of 2010 (HHFKA; P.L. 111-296), made a number of changes to the child nutrition programs. In some cases, these changes spurred debate during the law's implementation, particularly in regard to updated nutrition standards for school meals and snacks. On September 30, 2015, some of the authorities created by the HHFKA expired. Efforts to reauthorize the child nutrition programs in the 114th Congress, while not completed, considered several related issues and prompted further discussion about the programs. There were no substantial reauthorization attempts in the 115th Congress. Current issues discussed in this chapter include the following:

- Nutrition standards for school meals and snacks. The HHFKA required USDA to update the nutrition standards for school meals and other foods sold in schools. USDA issued final rules on these standards in 2012 and 2016, respectively. Some schools had difficulty implementing the nutrition standards, and USDA and Congress have taken actions to change certain parts of the standards related to whole grains, sodium, and milk.

- Offerings in the Fresh Fruit and Vegetable Program (FFVP). There have been debates recently over whether the FFVP should include processed and preserved fruits and vegetables, including canned, dried, and frozen items. Currently, statute permits only fresh offerings.
- "Buy American" requirements for school meals. The school meals programs' authorizing laws require schools to source foods domestically, with some exceptions, under Buy American requirements. Efforts both to tighten and loosen these requirements have been made in recent years. The enacted 2018 farm bill (P.L. 115-334) instructed USDA to "enforce full compliance" with the Buy American requirements and report to Congress within 180 days of enactment.
- Congregate feeding in summer meals. Under current law, children must consume summer meals on-site. This is known as the "congregate feeding" requirement. Starting in 2010, Congress funded demonstration projects, including the Summer Electronic Benefit Transfer (EBT) demonstration, to test alternatives to congregate feeding in summer meals. Congress has increased funding for Summer EBT in recent appropriations cycles and there have been discussions about whether to continue or expand the program.
- Implementation of the Community Eligibility Provision (CEP). The HHFKA created CEP, an option for qualifying schools, groups of schools, and school districts to offer free meals to all students. Because income-based applications for school meals are no longer required in schools adopting CEP, its implementation has created data issues for federal and state programs relying on free and reduced-price lunch eligibility data.
- Unpaid meal costs and "lunch shaming." The issue of students not paying for meals and schools' handling of these situations has received increasing attention. Some schools have adopted what some term as "lunch shaming" practices, including

throwing away a student's selected hot meal and providing a cold meal alternative when a student does not pay. Congress and USDA have taken actions recently to reduce instances of student nonpayment and stigmatization.

- Paid lunch pricing. One result of new requirements in the HHFKA was price increases for paid (full price) lunches in many schools. Attempts have been made—some successfully—to loosen these "paid lunch equity" requirements in recent years.

Chapter 2 - The child nutrition programs and the Special Supplemental Nutrition Program for Women, Infants, and Children (WIC) were last reauthorized in 2010. Some of the authorities created or extended in that law (Healthy, Hunger-Free Kids Act of 2010, P.L. 111-296) expired on September 30, 2015. However, the vast majority of program operations have continued with funding provided by appropriations acts. *Child nutrition reauthorization* refers to Congress's process of making changes, additions, and deletions to the permanent statutes that authorize the child nutrition programs, WIC, and related policies: (1) Richard B. Russell National School Lunch Act, (2) Child Nutrition Act, and sometimes (3) Section 32 of the Act of August 24, 1935. During the 114th Congress, committees of jurisdiction marked up bills but reauthorization was not completed (see CRS Report R44373, Tracking the Next Child Nutrition Reauthorization: An Overview).

Chapter 3 - The "child nutrition programs" refer to the U.S. Department of Agriculture's Food and Nutrition Service (USDA-FNS) programs that provide food for children in school or institutional settings. The best known programs, which serve the largest number of children, are the school meals programs: the National School Lunch Program (NSLP) and the School Breakfast Program (SBP). The child nutrition programs also include the Child and Adult Care Food Program (CACFP), which provides meals and snacks in day care and after school settings; the Summer Food Service Program (SFSP), which provides food during the summer months; the Special Milk Program (SMP), which supports milk for schools that do not participate in NSLP or SBP; and the Fresh Fruit and Vegetable Program (FFVP), which funds fruit and vegetable snacks in select elementary schools. Funding: The vast majority of the child nutrition programs account is considered mandatory spending, with trace amounts of discretionary funding for certain related activities. Referred to as open-ended, "appropriated entitlements," funding is provided through the annual appropriations process; however, the level of *spending* is controlled by benefit and eligibility criteria in federal law and dependent on the resulting levels of participation. Federal cash funding (in the form of per-meal reimbursements) and USDA commodity food support is guaranteed to schools and other providers based on the number of meals or snacks served and participant category (e.g., free meals for poor children get higher subsidies). Participation: The child nutrition programs serve children of varying ages and in different institutional settings. The NSLP and SBP have the broadest reach, serving qualifying children of all ages in school settings. Other child nutrition programs serve more-narrow populations. CACFP, for example, provides meals and snacks to children in early childhood and after-school settings among other venues. Programs generally provide some subsidy for all food served but a larger federal reimbursement for food served to children from low-income households. Administration: Responsibility for child nutrition programs is divided between the federal government, states, and localities. The state agency and type of local provider differs by program. In the NSLP and SBP, schools and school districts ("school food authorities") administer the program. Meanwhile, SFSP (and sometimes CACFP) uses a model in which sponsor organizations handle administrative responsibilities for a number of sites that serve meals. Reauthorization: The underlying laws covering the child nutrition programs were last reauthorized in the Healthy, Hunger-Free Kids Act of 2010 (HHFKA, P.L. 111-296, enacted December 13, 2010). This law made significant changes to child nutrition programs, including increasing federal financing for school lunches, expanding access to community eligibility and direct certification options for schools, and expanding eligibility options for home child care providers. The law also required an update to school meal nutrition guidelines as well as new guidelines for food served outside the meal programs (e.g., snacks sold in vending machines and cafeteria a la carte lines). Current Issues: The 114th Congress began but did not complete a 2016 child nutrition reauthorization, and there was no significant legislative activity with regard to reauthorization in the 115th Congress. However, the vast majority of operations and activities continue with funding provided by appropriations laws.

Chapter 4 - The SFSP, a federal nutrition assistance program, is intended to provide food to children in low-income areas during periods when area schools are closed for vacation. In the last decade, federal expenditures for SFSP have increased as the program has expanded, according to USDA data. GAO was asked to review the SFSP. This chapter examines (1) what is known about SFSP participation, (2) other programs that help feed low-income children over the summer, and (3) challenges, if any, in providing summer meals to children and the extent to which USDA provides assistance to address these challenges. GAO reviewed relevant federal laws, regulations, and guidance; analyzed USDA's SFSP data for fiscal years 2007 through 2016; surveyed state agencies responsible for administering the SFSP in 50 states and the District of Columbia; visited a nongeneralizable group of 3 states and 30 meal sites, selected based on Census data on child poverty rates and urban and rural locations; analyzed meal site data from the 3 states; and interviewed USDA, state and national organization officials, and SFSP providers, including sponsors and site operators.

Chapter 5 - This is an edited, reformatted and augmented version of United States Government Accountability Office; Testimony Before the Subcommittee on Early Childhood, Elementary, and Secondary Education, Committee on Education and the Workforce, House of Representatives; Accessible Version, Publication No. GAO-18-611T, dated July 17, 2018.

Chapter 6 - The Special Supplemental Nutrition Program for Women, Infants, and Children (WIC) provides nutrition-rich foods, nutrition education (including breastfeeding promotion and support), and health care and social services referrals to eligible low-income women, infants, and children. In FY2016, approximately 7.7 million people participated in WIC each month. WIC is authorized by the Child Nutrition Act, as is the related WIC Farmers' Market Nutrition Program (WIC FMNP). WIC, WIC FMNP, school meals, and the other child nutrition programs are typically reauthorized together; these programs were last reauthorized in the Healthy, Hunger-Free Kids Act of 2010 (P.L. 111-296). WIC's funding is discretionary, and the bulk of program funds are allocated via formula grant to state agencies for food costs and "Nutrition Services and Administration." In FY2016, there were 90 state agencies (50 states, District of Columbia, 5 U.S. territories, and 34 Indian Tribal Organizations). These agencies operate the program through local WIC agencies and clinics. The program obligated over $7 billion in federal funds in FY2014. WIC has a number of federal and state eligibility rules, including categorical, financial, and nutritional risk. Participants must fall into one of WIC's participant categories: pregnant, postpartum, and breastfeeding women; infants; or children (under five years of age). Financial eligibility is met if (1) a household has income at or below 185% of the federal poverty level, or (2) applicants receive benefits through Temporary Assistance for Needy Families (TANF), the Supplemental Nutrition Assistance Program (SNAP), Medicaid, or certain state programs. Households also must meet nutritional risk criteria and reside in the state of application. WIC provides participants with monthly benefits redeemable for specified foods to supplement their diets, as well as related nutrition and health services. WIC-eligible foods are laid out in federal regulation, and state agencies develop their own approved food lists within this framework. At the WIC clinic, participants are provided the benefits to redeem specific foods (food package) for the participant's category and individual nutritional needs. Major changes to the federal WIC food package regulations have been made in recent years; for some participant categories, the food package now includes a cash-value voucher redeemable for fruits and vegetables. One way that state agencies control WIC costs is through their approved foods lists. These lists usually include one brand of infant formula, as state agencies are required to control infant formula costs through competitive bidding for infant formula rebate contracts. In addition to providing food benefits, states are required to ensure that nutrition education, including breastfeeding promotion and drug abuse education, is available to all pregnant, postpartum, and breastfeeding participants in the program. Agencies also work to refer WIC participants to health services and other public programs, particularly Medicaid. Nearly all states administer their programs through a retail food delivery system, in which participants purchase foods at authorized retailers (vendors). Accordingly, many WIC policies at the federal and state levels pertain to vendor authorization and oversight as well as benefit redemption. Currently, most states distribute checks or vouchers for participants to purchase WIC foods at vendors; however, state agencies are increasingly transitioning to electronic benefit transfer (EBT), in part because the 2010 reauthorization law requires this transition by October 1, 2020. States authorize vendors for the program, considering factors like a vendor's inventory and capacity and geographic distribution of vendors. States also consider and monitor WIC vendors' pricing, as required by federal law, to help contain program costs.

Chapter 7 - This is an edited, reformatted and augmented version of United States Government Accountability Office; Congressional Committees, Publication No. GAO-18-125R, dated November 30, 2017.

Chapter 8 - SNAP is the largest federally funded nutrition assistance program. In fiscal year 2017, it provided about $63 billion in benefits. USDA and the states jointly administer SNAP and partner to address issues that affect program integrity, including improper payments and fraud. GAO has previously reported on various aspects of SNAP, including state SNAP E&T programs, improper payment rates, recipient fraud, and retailer trafficking. This testimony discusses GAO's prior and ongoing work on (1) SNAP E&T programs, including program participants, design, and USDA oversight, and (2) USDA's efforts to address SNAP program integrity, including improper payments, as well as recipient and retailer fraud. As part of its ongoing work on SNAP E&T programs, GAO analyzed E&T expenditures and participation data from fiscal years 2007 through 2016, the most recent data available; reviewed relevant research from USDA; and interviewed USDA and selected state and local officials. The prior work discussed in this testimony is based on four GAO products on E&T

programs (GAO-03-388), improper payments (GAO-16-708T), recipient fraud (GAO-14-641), and retailer trafficking (GAO-07-53). Information on the scope and methodology of our prior work is available in each product.

In: Child Nutrition Programs
Editor: Daniel D. Coleman
ISBN: 978-1-53615-764-2

Chapter 1

CHILD NUTRITION PROGRAMS: CURRENT ISSUES*

Kara Clifford Billings

ABSTRACT

The term *child nutrition programs* refers to several U.S. Department of Agriculture Food and Nutrition Service (USDA-FNS) programs that provide food for children in institutional settings. These include the school meals programs—the National School Lunch Program and School Breakfast Program—as well as the Child and Adult Care Food Program, Summer Food Service Program, Special Milk Program, and Fresh Fruit and Vegetable Program.

The most recent child nutrition reauthorization, the Healthy, Hunger-Free Kids Act of 2010 (HHFKA; P.L. 111-296), made a number of changes to the child nutrition programs. In some cases, these changes spurred debate during the law's implementation, particularly in regard to updated nutrition standards for school meals and snacks. On September 30, 2015, some of the authorities created by the HHFKA expired. Efforts to reauthorize the child nutrition programs in the 114th Congress, while

* This is an edited, reformatted and augmented version of Congressional Research Service, Publication No. R45486, dated January 31, 2019.

not completed, considered several related issues and prompted further discussion about the programs. There were no substantial reauthorization attempts in the 115th Congress.

Current issues discussed in this chapter include the following:

- Nutrition standards for school meals and snacks. The HHFKA required USDA to update the nutrition standards for school meals and other foods sold in schools. USDA issued final rules on these standards in 2012 and 2016, respectively. Some schools had difficulty implementing the nutrition standards, and USDA and Congress have taken actions to change certain parts of the standards related to whole grains, sodium, and milk.
- Offerings in the Fresh Fruit and Vegetable Program (FFVP). There have been debates recently over whether the FFVP should include processed and preserved fruits and vegetables, including canned, dried, and frozen items. Currently, statute permits only fresh offerings.
- "Buy American" requirements for school meals. The school meals programs' authorizing laws require schools to source foods domestically, with some exceptions, under Buy American requirements. Efforts both to tighten and loosen these requirements have been made in recent years. The enacted 2018 farm bill (P.L. 115-334) instructed USDA to "enforce full compliance" with the Buy American requirements and report to Congress within 180 days of enactment.
- Congregate feeding in summer meals. Under current law, children must consume summer meals on-site. This is known as the "congregate feeding" requirement. Starting in 2010, Congress funded demonstration projects, including the Summer Electronic Benefit Transfer (EBT) demonstration, to test alternatives to congregate feeding in summer meals. Congress has increased funding for Summer EBT in recent appropriations cycles and there have been discussions about whether to continue or expand the program.
- Implementation of the Community Eligibility Provision (CEP). The HHFKA created CEP, an option for qualifying schools, groups of schools, and school districts to offer free meals to all students. Because income-based applications for school meals are no longer required in schools adopting CEP, its implementation has created data issues for federal and state programs relying on free and reduced-price lunch eligibility data.
- Unpaid meal costs and "lunch shaming." The issue of students not paying for meals and schools' handling of these situations has received increasing attention. Some schools have adopted what some term as "lunch shaming" practices, including throwing away a

student's selected hot meal and providing a cold meal alternative when a student does not pay. Congress and USDA have taken actions recently to reduce instances of student nonpayment and stigmatization.

- Paid lunch pricing. One result of new requirements in the HHFKA was price increases for paid (full price) lunches in many schools. Attempts have been made—some successfully—to loosen these "paid lunch equity" requirements in recent years.

INTRODUCTION

The term *child nutrition programs* refers to several U.S. Department of Agriculture Food and Nutrition Service (USDA-FNS) programs that provide food to children in institutional settings. The largest are the National School Lunch Program (NSLP) and School Breakfast Program (SBP), which subsidize free, reduced-price, and full-price meals in participating schools.[1] Also operating in schools, the Fresh Fruit and Vegetable Program provides funding for fruit and vegetable snacks in participating elementary schools, and the Special Milk Program provides support for milk in schools that do not participate in NSLP or SBP. Other child nutrition programs include the Child and Adult Care Food Program, which provides meals and snacks in child care and after-school settings, and the Summer Food Service Program, which provides food during the summer months.[2]

The child nutrition programs were last reauthorized by the Healthy, Hunger-Free Kids Act of 2010 (HHFKA, P.L. 111-296). On September 30, 2015, some of the authorities created or extended by the HHFKA

---

[1] These three meal categories are subsidized by the federal government in increasing amounts. For the reimbursement rates for school year (SY) 2018-2019, see USDA-FNS, "National School Lunch, Special Milk, and School Breakfast Programs, National Average Payments/Maximum Reimbursement Rates," 83 *Federal Register* 34105, July, 19, 2018, https://www.federalregister.gov/documents/2018/07/19/2018-15465/national-school-lunch-special-milk-and-schoolbreakfast-programs-national-average-paymentsmaximum.

[2] The Special Supplemental Nutrition Program for Women, Infants, and Children (WIC) is typically reauthorized with the child nutrition programs but is not considered a child nutrition program because it is not administered in institutional settings. For more information on WIC, see CRS Report R44115, *A Primer on WIC: The Special Supplemental Nutrition Program for Women, Infants, and Children*.

expired. However, these expirations had a minimal impact on program operations, as the child nutrition programs have continued with funding provided by annual appropriations acts.[3]

In the 114th Congress, lawmakers began but did not complete child nutrition reauthorization, which refers to the process of reauthorizing and potentially making changes to multiple permanent statutes—the Richard B. Russell National School Lunch Act, the Child Nutrition Act, and sometimes Section 32 of the Act of August 24, 1935. Both committees of jurisdiction—the Senate Committee on Agriculture, Nutrition, and Forestry and the House Committee on Education and the Workforce—reported reauthorization legislation (S. 3136 and H.R. 5003, respectively). This legislation died at the end of the 114th Congress, as is the case for any bill that has not yet passed both chambers and been sent to the President at the end of a Congress. There were no significant child nutrition reauthorization efforts in the 115th Congress; however, 2018 farm bill proposals and the final enacted bill included a few provisions related to child nutrition programs.

The implementation of the HHFKA, child nutrition reauthorization efforts in the 114th Congress, and the child nutrition-related topics raised during 2018 farm bill negotiations have raised issues that may be relevant for Congress in future reauthorization efforts or other policymaking opportunities. These issues often relate to the content and type of foods served in schools: for example, the nutritional quality of foods and whether foods are domestically sourced. Other issues relate to access, including alternatives to on-site consumption in summer meals and implementation of the Community Eligibility Provision, an option to provide free meals to all students in certain schools. Stakeholders in these issues commonly include school food authorities (SFAs; school food service departments that

[3] Most of the child nutrition programs are "appropriated entitlements," meaning that the authorizing law sets a level of spending that Congress must fulfill through an appropriation. In FY2016, FY2017, and FY2018, enacted annual appropriation laws and continuing resolutions enabled the child nutrition programs to continue operating. For more information, see CRS In Focus IF10266, *An Introduction to Child Nutrition Reauthorization*.

generally operate at the school district level), hunger and nutrition-focused advocacy organizations, and food industry organizations, among others.

This chapter provides an overview of these and other current issues in the child nutrition programs. It does not cover every issue, but rather provides a high-level review of some recent issues raised by Congress and/or program stakeholders, drawing examples from legislative proposals in the 114th and 115th Congresses.

Table 1. Child Nutrition Programs' Authorizing Laws and Regulations

Program	Authorizing Statutes	Regulations
National School Lunch Program (NSLP)	Richard B. Russell National School Lunch Act (42 U.S.C. 1751 et seq.)	7 C.F.R. 210 et seq.
School Breakfast Program (SBP)	Child Nutrition Act, Section 4 (42 U.S.C. 1773)	7 C.F.R. 220 et seq.
Child and Adult Care Food Program (CACFP)	Richard B. Russell National School Lunch Act, Section 17 (42 U.S.C. 1766)	7 C.F.R. 226 et seq.
Summer Food Service Program (SFSP)	Richard B. Russell National School Lunch Act, Section 13 (42 U.S.C. 1761)	7 C.F.R. 225 et seq.
Special Milk Program (SMP)	Child Nutrition Act, Section 3 (42 U.S.C. 1772)	7 C.F.R. 215 et seq.
Fresh Fruit and Vegetable Program (FFVP)	Richard B. Russell National School Lunch Act, Section 19 (42 U.S.C. 1769[a])	n/a[a]

Source: Compiled by CRS.

[a] FFVP currently operates according to statute and USDA guidance. USDA-FNS issued a proposed rule in 2012 to codify statutory requirements in regulations, but a final rule has not been published.

Current Issues

Nutrition Standards for School Meals and Snacks Background

School meals must meet certain requirements to be eligible for federal reimbursement, including nutritional requirements. These nutrition standards were last updated following the enactment of the HHFKA, which created a timeline for USDA to update the standards for school meals and create new nutrition standards for "competitive" foods (e.g., foods sold in vending machines, a lacarte lines, and snack bars).[4] For the most part, the precise nutritional requirements were written in regulations, not the HHFKA. The law required USDA to issue proposed regulations for competitive foods standards within one year after enactment and for school meals standards within 18 months after enactment. The law also provided increased federal subsidies (6 cents per lunch) for schools meeting the new requirements and funding for technical assistance. The nutrition standards were championed by then-First Lady Michelle Obama through her "Let's Move" initiative.[5]

USDA-FNS published the final rule for school meals in January 2012 and the final rule for competitive foods in July 2016.[6] As required by law, the nutrition standards were based on the Dietary Guidelines for Americans and recommendations from the Institute of Medicine (now the Health and Medicine Division of the National Academies).[7] For school meals, the updated standards increased the amount of fruits, vegetables, and whole grains in school lunches and breakfasts.[8] They also instituted limits on calories, sodium, whole grains, and proteins in meals and restricted milk to low-fat (unflavored) and fat-free (flavored or unflavored) varieties. Other requirements included a provision that senior high school students must select a half-serving of fruits or vegetables with

---

[4] Section 201 and Section 208 of P.L. 111-296.

[5] See, for example, Nia-Malika Henderson, "President Obama signs child nutrition bill, a priority for first lady," *Washington Post*, December 13, 2010, http://www.washingtonpost.com/wp-dyn/content/article/2010/12/13/ AR2010121302407.html; archived White House website, "Let's Move, Healthy Schools," https://letsmove.obamawhitehouse.archives.gov/healthy-schools.

[6] USDA-FNS, "Nutrition Standards in the National School Lunch and School Breakfast Programs," 77 *Federal Register* 17, January 26, 2012, https://www.federalregister.gov/documents/2012/01/26/2012-1010/nutrition-standardsin-the-national-school-lunch-and-school-breakfast-programs; USDA-FNS, "National School Lunch Program and School Breakfast Program: Nutrition Standards for All Foods Sold in School as Required by the Healthy, Hunger-Free Kids Act of 2010; Final Rule," 81 *Federal Register* 50131, July 29, 2016, https://www.federalregister.gov/documents/ 2016/07/29/2016-17227/national-school-lunch-program-and-school-breakfast-program-nutrition-standards-for-allfoods-sold-in. For current nutritional requirements, see 7 C.F.R. 210.10 for the NSLP and 7 C.F.R. 220.8 for the SBP.

[7] Section 201, Section 208, and Section 441 of P.L. 111-296.

[8] See USDA-FNS, Comparison of Previous and New Regulatory Requirements, https://fns-prod.azureedge.net/sites/ default/files/cn/comparison.pdf

a reimbursable meal.[9] Similarly, the nutrition standards for competitive foods limited calories, sodium, and fat in foods sold outside of meals, among other requirements.[10] The standards applied only to nonmeal foods and beverages sold *during the school day* (defined as midnight until 30 minutes after dismissal) and include some exceptions for fundraisers.

Implementation and Changes

The meal standards began phasing in during school year (SY) 2012-2013, and the competitive foods standards took effect in SY2014-2015.[11] However, sodium limits and certain whole grain requirements for school meals were scheduled to phase in over multiple school years.[12] Some schools experienced challenges implementing the changes, reporting difficulty obtaining whole grain and low-sodium products, issues with student acceptance of foods, reduced participation, increased costs, and increased food waste. These accounts were shared in news stories and by the School Nutrition Association (SNA), a national, nonprofit professional and advocacy organization representing school nutrition professionals.[13]

---

[9] This is commonly known as the "offer versus serve" requirement because it can result in schools having to serve, rather than offer, a half-serving of fruits or vegetables to high school students.

[10] Related information is available at the USDA-FNS website: https://www.fns.usda.gov/school-meals/tools-schoolsfocusing-smart-snacks.

[11] For the original implementation schedule based on the January 2012 final rule, see USDA-FNS, Implementation Timeline, .http://www.fns.usda.gov/sites/default/files/implementation_timeline.pdf. Most of the lunch requirements took effect in SY2012-2013, while most breakfast requirements took effect in SY2013-2014.

[12] Ibid.

[13] For examples of news coverage, see B. Wood, *Students, parents, educators displeased with new school lunch standards*, Deseret News, September 27, 2012, https://www.deseretnews.com/article/865563339/Students-parentseducators-displeased-with-new-school-lunch-standards.html; and L. Lopez, *"We're Still Hungry!" Student Lunches Leave Stomachs Rumbling*, NBCLA, September 26, 2012, https://www.nbclosangeles.com/news/local/Los-AngelesUnified-School-District-LAUSD-Nutrition-School-Lunch-No-Kid-Hungry-171439851.html. Also see School Nutrition Association, *Stories from the Frontlines: School Cafeteria Professionals Discuss Challenges with New Standards*, May 28, 2014, https://schoolnutrition.org/5—News-and-Publications/2—Press-Releases/Press-Releases/Stories-from-theFrontlines—School-Cafeteria-Professionals-Discuss-Challenges-with-New-Standards/.

Studies by the U.S. Government Accountability Office and USDA confirmed that many of these issues were present in SY2012-2013 and SY2013-2014, the first two years of implementation.[14] SNA advocated for certain changes to the standards, while other groups called for maintaining the standards, arguing that they were necessary for children's health and that implementation challenges were easing with time.[15]

In January 2014, USDA removed weekly limits on grains and protein.[16] Then, in the FY2015, FY2016, and FY2017 appropriations laws, Congress enacted provisions that loosened the milk, whole grain, and/or sodium requirements from SY2015-2016 through SY2017-2018.[17] USDA implemented similar changes for SY2018-2019 in an interim final rule.[18] In December 2018, USDA published a final rule that indefinitely changes these three aspects of the standards starting in SY2019-2020.[19]

---

[14] U.S. Government Accountability Office (GAO), *Implementing Nutrition Changes Was Challenging and Clarification of Oversight Requirements Is Needed*, January 2014, https://www.gao.gov/assets/670/660427.pdf; Standing et al., *Special Nutrition Program Operations Study: State and School Food Authority Policies and Practices for School Meals Programs School Year 2012-13*, prepared by Westat for USDA-FNS, October 2016; J. Murdoch et al., *Special Nutrition Program Operations Study, SY 2013-14 Report*, prepared by 2M Research Services, 2016; GAO, *USDA Has Efforts Underway to Help Address Ongoing Challenges Implementing Changes in Nutrition Standards*, September 2015, https://www.gao.gov/assets/680/672477.pdf. Numerous studies have examined the efficacy of the nutrition standards in these and more recent school years in terms of a number of programmatic outcomes, including participation rates, food waste, and nutritional quality. It is beyond the scope of this chapter to review this entire body of literature.

[15] For example, see School Nutrition Association, *2014 Position Paper on Federal Child Nutrition Programs*, https://schoolnutrition.org/uploadedFiles/Legislation_and_Policy/SNA_Policy_Resources/SNA2014PositionPaper.pdf; and archived USDA-FNS web page, *Support for Healthy Meals Standards Continues to Grow*, May 2014, https://www.fns.usda.gov/pressrelease/2014/012714.

[16] USDA-FNS, "Certification of Compliance With Meal Requirements for the National School Lunch Program Under the Healthy, Hunger-Free Kids Act of 2010," 79 *Federal Register* 325, January 3, 2014, https://www.federalregister.gov/documents/2014/01/03/2013-31433/certification-of-compliance-with-mealrequirements-for-the-national-school-lunch-program-under-the.

[17] P.L. 113-235, P.L. 114-113, and P.L. 115-31.

[18] USDA-FNS, "Child Nutrition Programs: Flexibilities for Milk, Whole Grains, and Sodium Requirements; Interim Final Rule," 82 *Federal Register* 56703, November 30, 2017, https://www.federalregister.gov/documents/2017/11/30/ 2017-25799/child-nutrition-programs-flexibilities-for-milk-whole-grains-and-sodium-requirements.

[19] USDA-FNS, "Child Nutrition Programs: Flexibilities for Milk, Whole Grains, and Sodium Requirements: Final Rule," 83 *Federal Register* 63775, December 12, 2018,

Specifically, the rule

- allows all SFAs to offer flavored, low-fat (1%) milk as part of school meals and as beverages sold in schools,[20] and requires unflavored milk to be offered alongside flavored milk in school meals;
- requires SFAs to adhere to a 50% whole grain-rich requirement (the original regulations required 100% whole grain-rich starting in SY2014-2015);[21] states may make exemptions to allow SFAs to offer nonwhole grain-rich products; and
- maintains Target 1 sodium limits from SY2019-2020 through SY2023-2024, implements Target 2 limits starting in SY2024-2025 and thereafter, and eliminates Target 3 limits (the strictest target).[22]

Table 2 provides a timeline from the 2012 final rule to the 2018 final rule, showing the ways in which milk, whole grain, and sodium requirements have been modified over time. Apart from these changes, the nutrition standards for school meals remain largely intact. The changes to the milk requirements also affect other beverages sold in schools; otherwise, the nutrition standards for competitive foods have not been changed substantially.

---

https://www.federalregister.gov/documents/2018/12/12/2018- 26762/child-nutrition-programs-flexibilities-for-milk-whole-grains-and-sodium-requirements.

[20] The final rule also allows flavored, low-fat milk to be served to children ages six and older in CACFP and SMP.

[21] USDA-FNS, *Grain Requirements for the National School Lunch Program and School Breakfast Program*, SP 30- 2012, April 26, 2012, https://fns-prod.azureedge.net/sites/default/files/cn/SP30-2012os.pdf. "Whole grain-rich" products must contain at least 50% whole-grains, and the remaining grain, if any, must be enriched.

[22] The sodium targets set incrementally stricter weekly caps on sodium in school meals based on a student's grade level. The standards included three incrementally stricter targets that were to phase in over time (Target 1, Target 2, and Target 3). For example, for high school students, school lunches must contain ≤1,420 milligrams (mg) of sodium under Target 1, ≤1,080 mg under Target 2, and ≤740 mg under Target 3, on average over the school week.

Table 2. Legislative and Regulatory Changes to the Milk, Whole Grain, and Sodium Requirements for School Meals (2012-2018)

Policy Provision	Milk	Whole Grains	Sodium
USDA-FNS January 2012 final rule[a]	Required flavored milk to be fat-free and unflavored milk to be low-fat (1%) or fat-free by SY2012-2013.	Required 50% of grains to be whole-grain rich by SY2012-2013 for lunches ad by SY2013-2014 for breakfasts; required 100% whole grain-rich by SY2014-2015.	Created maximum weekly levels of sodium for breakfasts and lunches based on a student's grade level. Scheduled Target 1 limits for SY2014-2015, Target 2 limits for SY2017-2018, and Target 3 limits for SY2022-2023.
FY2015 appropriation (§§751 and 752 of P.L.113-235)	n/a	Required USDA to allow states to exempt SFAs demonstrating hardship from the 100% whole grain requirement from December 2014 through SY2015-2016. Exempted SFAs must comply with the 50% requirement.	Postponed reductions in sodium below Target 1 indefinitely ("until the latest scientific research establishes the reduction is beneficial for children").
FY2016 appropriation (§733 of P.L. 114-113)	n/a	Extended exemptions through SY2016-2017.	Same language as FY2015.
FY2017 appropriation (§747 of P.L. 115-31)	Required USDA to allow states to grant hardship based exemptions to SFAs to offer flavored low-fat (1%) milk from May 2017 through SY2017-2018.	Extended exemptions through SY2017-2018.	Retained Target 1 through SY2017-2018.
USDA-FNS November 2017 interim final rule[b]	Allowed all SFAs to offer flavored low-fat (1%) milk in SY2018-2019.	Extended exemptions through SY2018-2019.	Retained Target 1 through SY2018-2019.

Policy Provision	Milk	Whole Grains	Sodium
USDA-FNS December 2018 final rule[c]	Allows all SFAs to offer flavored low-fat (1%) milk in SY2019-2020 and thereafter.	Institutes 50% whole grain requirement for all SFAs starting in SY2019-2020 and thereafter. Allows states to grant exemptions to SFAs to offer grains that are not whole-grain rich.	Retains Target 1 in SY2019-2020 through SY2023-2024, implements Target 2 starting in SY2024-2025 and thereafter, and eliminates Target 3.

Source: Compiled by CRS.

Notes: n/a indicates that the law did not include pertinent content. The FY2017 appropriation was enacted shortly after the November 2017 interim final rule but is presented before it in this table because of the school years that each policy affected. Not shown are (1) the FY2012 appropriations act, which retained Target 1 indefinitely and prohibited the establishment of any whole grain requirements that did not define "whole grain," and (2) USDA guidance and regulations that lifted weekly maximums on whole grains starting in 2012.

a. USDA-FNS, "Nutrition Standards in the National School Lunch and School Breakfast Programs," 77 *Federal Register* 17, January 26, 2012, https://www.federalregister.gov/ documents/2012/01/26/2012-1010/nutritionstandards-in-the-national-school-lunch-and-school-breakfast-programs.

b. USDA-FNS, "Child Nutrition Programs: Flexibilities for Milk, Whole Grains, and Sodium Requirements; Interim Final Rule," 82 *Federal Register* 56703, November 30, 2017, https://www.federalregister.gov/ documents/2017/11/30/2017-25799/child-nutrition-programs-flexibilities-for-milk-whole-grains-and-sodiumrequirements.

c. USDA-FNS, "Child Nutrition Programs: Flexibilities for Milk, Whole Grains, and Sodium Requirements: Final Rule," 83 *Federal Register* 63775, December 12, 2018, https://www.federalregister.gov/documents/2018/ 12/12/2018-26762/child-nutrition-programs-flexibilities-for-milk-whole-grains-and-sodium-requirements.

Other Proposals

Legislative proposals related to the nutrition standards were considered in the 115th Congress. For example, the House-passed version of 2018 farm bill (one version of H.R. 2) would have required USDA to review and revise the nutrition standards for school meals and competitive foods. According to the bill, the revisions would have had to ensure that the standards, particularly those related to milk, "(1) are based on research based on school-age children; (2) do not add costs in addition to the reimbursements required to carry out the school lunch program ... and (3) maintain healthy meals for students."[23] This provision was not included in the enacted bill.

Child nutrition reauthorization proposals in the House and Senate during the 114th Congress also would have altered the nutrition standards. The House committee's proposal (H.R. 5003) would have required USDA to review the school meal standards at least once every three years and revise them as necessary, following certain criteria.[24] In addition, under the proposal, fundraisers by student groups/organizations would no longer have had to meet the competitive food standards and any foods served as part of a federally reimbursable meal would have been allowed to be sold a la carte.[25] The Senate committee's proposal (S. 3136) would have required USDA to revise the whole grain and sodium requirements for school meals within 90 days after enactment. Although not included in the proposal itself, negotiations between the Senate committee, the White House,

USDA, and the School Nutrition Association resulted in an agreement that these revisions, if enacted, would have reduced the 100% whole grain-rich requirement to 80% and delayed the Target 2 sodium requirement for two years.[26]

"Fresh" in the Fresh Fruit and Vegetable Program (FFVP)

Under current law, fruit and vegetable snacks served in FFVP must be fresh.[27] According to USDA guidance, fresh refers to foods "in their

---

[23] Section 4205 of H.R. 2 (as engrossed in the House on June 21, 2018).

[24] The Secretary of Agriculture, with consultation from school stakeholders, would have been required to certify that certain requirements were met, including that the regulations were age-appropriate, did not increase the costs of implementing the school meals programs, and did not discourage students from participating in the school meals programs.

[25] For more information, see CRS Report R44373, *Tracking the Next Child Nutrition Reauthorization: An Overview*.

[26] The SNA posted a January 15, 2016, statement of the terms of the agreement at https://schoolnutrition.org/News/AgreementReachedOnSchoolNutritionStandards/. The terms were also discussed in a colloquy between Ranking Member Debbie Stabenow and Senator John Hoeven during the committee's markup.

[27] Section 19 of the Richard B. Russell National School Lunch Act (42 U.S.C. 1769a).

natural state and without additives."[28] In recent years, some have advocated for the inclusion of frozen, dried, canned, and other types of fruits and vegetables in the program, while others have advocated for continuing to maintain only fresh products.[29] Stakeholders on both sides include agricultural producers and processors.

The 2014 farm bill (Section 4214 of P.L. 113-79) funded a pilot project that incorporated canned, dried, and frozen (CDF) fruits and vegetables in FFVP in a limited number of states. USDA selected schools in four states (Alaska, Delaware, Kansas, and Maine) that reported difficulty obtaining, storing, and/or preparing fresh fruits and vegetables. According to the final (2017) evaluation, 56% of the pilot schools chose to incorporate CDF fruits and vegetables during an average week of the demonstration.[30] Schools most often introduced dried and canned fruits, which resulted in decreased vegetable offerings and increased fruit offerings in the FFVP. However, there was no significant impact on students' vegetable consumption, while fruit consumption declined on FFVP snack days (likely because students consumed a smaller quantity of fruit when it was dried or canned). There was also no significant impact on student participation. Student satisfaction with FFVP decreased slightly during the pilot, parents' responses to the pilot were mixed, and school administrators (who opted into the pilot) generally favored the changes.

Legislative proposals to change FFVP offerings on a more permanent basis have also been considered. For example, in the 115th Congress, the House version of H.R. 2 would have allowed CDF and puréed forms of fruits and vegetables in FFVP and removed "fresh" from the program name. This provision was not included in the enacted bill. In the 114th

---

[28] USDA-FNS, *Fresh Fruit and Vegetable Program: A Handbook for Schools*, December 2010, p. 15, https://fnsprod.azureedge.net/sites/default/files/handbook.pdf.

[29] American Frozen Food Institute, *House Support Expansion Letter of FFVP in CNR,* April 7, 2016, http://www.affi.org/assets/resources/public/house-support-letter-expansion-of-ffvp-in-cnr-april-2016_2.pdf; United Fresh, *National Produce Leaders FFVP Letter to House,* April 21, 2016, https://www.unitedfresh.org/content/uploads/ 2016/05/National-Produce-Leaders-FFVP-Letter-to-House.pdf.

[30] USDA-FNS, Evaluation of the Pilot Project for Canned, Frozen, or Dried Fruits and Vegetables in the Fresh Fruit and Vegetable Program (FFVP-CFD): Volume I: Report, prepared by Mathematica Policy Research, January 2017, https://fns-prod. azureedge.net/sites/default/files/ops/FFVP-CFD.pdf.

Congress, child nutrition reauthorization legislation in the House (H.R. 5003) included a similar proposal to allow participating schools to serve "all forms" of fruits and vegetables as well as tree nuts. The Senate committee's proposal (S. 3136) would have provided temporary hardship exemptions for schools with limited storage and preparation facilities or limited access to fresh fruits and vegetables that would have allowed them to serve CDF fruits and vegetables in FFVP. Such schools would have to transition to 100% fresh products over time.

"Buy American" in School Meals Programs

Schools participating in the National School Lunch Program (NSLP) and/or School Breakfast Program (SBP) must comply with federal requirements related to sourcing foods domestically. These requirements are outlined in the school meals programs' authorizing laws and clarified in USDA guidance.

Under the Buy American requirements, schools participating in the NSLP and/or SBP in the 48 contiguous states must purchase "domestic commodities or products ... to the maximum extent practicable."[31] Statute defines "domestic commodities or products" as those that are both produced and processed substantially in the United States. Accompanying conference report language elaborated that "processed substantially" means the product is processed in the United States and contains over 51% domestically grown ingredients, and this definition is also included

[31] Section 12(n) of the Richard B. Russell National School Lunch Act (42 U.S.C. 1760(n)). Alaska is exempt and Hawaii and Puerto Rico are subject to separate but related requirements.

in USDA guidance (discussed below).[32] USDA regulations essentially restate the statutory requirement.[33]

USDA has issued guidance on how SFAs and state agencies should implement the Buy American requirements. The most recent guidance (as of the date of this chapter) was published in a June 2017 memorandum.[34] According to USDA-FNS guidance, the Buy American requirements apply to any foods purchased with funds from the nonprofit school food service account, whether or not they are federal funds (children's paid lunch fees, for example, also go into the nonprofit school food service account).[35] The guidance encourages SFAs to integrate Buy American into their procurement processes; for example, by monitoring the USDA catalog for appropriate products and placing Buy American language in solicitations, contracts, and other procurement documents. The guidance explains that SFAs are permitted to make exceptions to the Buy American requirements on a limited basis when a product "is not produced or manufactured in the U.S. in sufficient and reasonably available quantities of a satisfactory quality" or when "competitive bids reveal the costs of a U.S. product are significantly higher than the non-domestic product."[36] SFAs must interpret when this is the case and document any exceptions they make. SFAs may also request a waiver from the requirements for a product that does not meet these criteria. State agencies must review SFAs' compliance with the Buy American requirements, including any exceptions an SFA has made, and take corrective action when necessary.

The enacted 2018 farm bill (Section 4207 of P.L. 115-334) included a provision requiring USDA to "enforce full compliance" with the Buy

---

[32] U.S. Congress, Conference Committee, William F. Goodling Child Nutrition Reauthorization Act of 1998, conference report to accompany H.R. 3874, 105th Cong., 2nd sess., H.Rept. 105-786 (Washington, DC: GPO, 1998), p. 38. According to USDA guidance, more than 51% means that more than 51% of a product's "food components," as defined in 7 C.F.R. 210.2 (meats/meat alternatives, grains, vegetables, fruits, and fluid milk) and as measured by weight or volume must be domestically grown in the United States or U.S. territories.

[33] 7 C.F.R. 210.21 and 7 C.F.R. 220.16.

[34] USDA-FNS, *Compliance with and Enforcement of the Buy American Provision in the National School Lunch Program*, SP 38-2017, June 30, 2017, https://fns-prod.azureedge.net/sites/default/files/cn/SP38-2017os.pdf.

[35] Ibid.

[36] Ibid, p. 3.

American requirements and "ensure that States and school food authorities fully understand their responsibilities" within 180 days of enactment. In addition, the bill requires USDA to submit a report to Congress by the 180-day deadline on actions taken and plans to comply with the provision. The provision clarifies the definition of domestic products for the purposes of USDA's enforcement, stating that domestic products are those that are "processed in the United States and substantially contain ... meats, vegetables, fruits, and other agricultural commodities" produced in the United States, the District of Columbia, Puerto Rico, or any territory or possession of the United States, or "fish harvested" in the Exclusive Economic Zone or by a U.S.-flagged vessel. The provision in the enacted bill amended a related provision in the Senate-passed version of the farm bill.[37]

Proponents of stricter requirements have cited economic and food safety reasons for domestic sourcing and expressed particular concern over sourcing from China.[38] Others have argued for maintaining or increasing schools' discretion in food procurement, arguing that high-quality domestic options are not always available or cost-effective.[39]

Alternatives to Congregate Feeding in Summer Meals

Under current law, summer meals are generally provided in "congregate" or group settings where children come to eat while supervised. These meals are provided through the Summer Food Service Program (SFSP) and the National School Lunch Program's Summer

---

[37] Section 12622 of H.R. 2 (as passed in the Senate on June 28, 2018).

[38] See, for example, National Council of Farmer Cooperatives et al., *Enforcement of Buy American Provision Letter,* December 2015, http://ncfc.org/letter/enforcement-of-buy-american-provision/; Murphy.senate.gov, *Murphy, Feinstein, Boxer Call On Schools to Buy American & Support Local Farmers*, https://www.murphy.senate.gov/newsroom/press-releases/murphy-feinstein-boxer-call-on-schools-to-buy-american-and-support-local-farmers; Lamalfa.house.gov, *LaMalfa and Garamendi Introduce the "American Food for American Schools" Act*, March 1, 2017, https://lamalfa.house.gov/media-center/press-releases/lamalfa-and-garamendi-introduce-the-american-food-foramerican-schools.

[39] H. Bottemiller Evich, *USDA's enforcement of 'Buy American' regulations strains school-meal programs*, PoliticoPro, March 5, 2018.

Seamless Option (SSO).[40] In recent years, policymakers have weighed different proposals and tested alternatives to congregate meals in SFSP and SSO. Some of these alternatives focus on rural areas, which may face particular barriers to onsite consumption of summer meals. According to a May 2018 study by the U.S. Government Accountability Office, states commonly reported that reaching children in rural areas was "very" or "extremely" challenging in SFSP.[41]

Summer EBT Demonstration

The 2010 Agriculture Appropriations Act (Section 749(g) of P.L. 111-80) provided $85 million in discretionary funding for "demonstration projects to develop and test methods of providing access to food for children in urban and rural areas during the summer months." One of these is the Summer Electronic Benefit Transfer for Children (SEBTC or Summer EBT) project, which began in summer 2011 and has continued each summer since (as of the date of this chapter) in a limited number of states and Indian Tribal Organizations.[42] The project provides electronic food benefits to households with children eligible for free or reduced-price school meals. Depending on the site and year, either $30 or $60 per month is provided on an electronic benefits transfer (EBT) card for the Special Supplemental Nutrition Program for Women, Infants, and Children (WIC) or Supplemental Nutrition Assistance Program (SNAP). Participants in jurisdictions providing benefits through SNAP can redeem benefits for SNAP-eligible foods at any SNAP-authorized retailer, while participants in the WIC EBT jurisdictions are limited to the smaller set of WIC-eligible foods at WIC-authorized retailers.[43]

---

[40] To learn more about these programs, see CRS Report R43783, *School Meals Programs and Other USDA Child Nutrition Programs: A Primer*.

[41] U.S. Government Accountability Office (GAO), *Summer Meals: Actions Needed to Improve Participation Estimates and Address Program Challenges*, May 2018, pp. 23-30, https://www.gao.gov/assets/700/692193.pdf.

[42] USDA-FNS, *Summer Electronic Benefit Transfer for Children (SEBTC)*, https://www.fns.usda.gov/ops/summerelectronic-benefit-transfer-children-sebtc.

[43] Collins et al., *Summer Electronic Benefit Transfer for Children (SEBTC) Demonstration: Summary Report*, prepared by Abt Associates Inc. for USDA-FNS, May 2016, p.5, https://fns-prod.azureedge.net/sites/default/files/ops/ sebtcfinalreport.pdf. Also see USDA-FNS, *WIC Food Packages - Regulatory Requirements for WIC-Eligible Foods,* April 2018,

An evaluation of Summer EBT was conducted from FY2011 through FY2013.[44] The study, which used a random assignment design, found a significant decline in the prevalence of very low food security among participants (9.5% of control group children experienced very low food security compared to 6.4% in the Summer EBT group).[45] It also showed improvements in children's consumption of fruits, vegetables, and whole grains. Both the WIC and SNAP models showed increased consumption, but increases were greater at sites operating the WIC model.[46]

Congress has provided subsequent funding for Summer EBT projects (see Table 3). Most recently, the FY2018 appropriations act (P.L. 115-141) provided $28 million for the Summer EBT demonstration. Awardees for summer 2017 were Connecticut, Delaware, Michigan, Missouri, Nevada, Oregon, Virginia, and the Chickasaw and Cherokee nations.[47] For summer 2018, USDA also awarded grants to Tennessee and Texas.[48] Many of these jurisdictions participated in Summer EBT in previous summers as well. In October 2018, USDA-FNS announced a new strategy for determining grant recipients in FY2019, stating that the agency will prioritize new

---

https://www.fns.usda.gov/wic/wic-food-packages-regulatory-requirements-wic-eligible-foods.

[44] The first year—the proof-of-concept year—was evaluated to test the feasibility of the EBT delivery system and to prepare for full implementation in demonstration sites for the following year. The second year—the full implementation year—evaluated the impact of SEBTC on improving children's food security and nutritional status in the summer time. Finally, the third year compared the impact of two benefit levels, $60 and $30, to determine the effect of different benefit levels on improving food security and nutritional status. Final reports and status reports to Congress are available on the USDA-FNS website, http://www.fns.usda.gov/ops/summer-electronic-benefit-transfer-childrensebtc.

[45] Collins et al., *Summer Electronic Benefits Transfer for Children (SEBTC) Demonstration: Evaluation Findings for the Full Implementation Year,* prepared by Abt Associates, Mathematica Policy Research, and Maximus (Alexandria, VA: USDA-FNS, 2013), p. 105. Very Low Food Security (VLFS) is the lowest of four levels of food security; USDA defines it as "At times during the year, eating patterns of one or more household members were disrupted and food intake reduced because the household lacked money and other resources for food." Improvements in VLFS varied significantly between Summer EBT sites.

[46] Ibid, p. 124.

[47] USDA-FNS, *USDA Announces Summer EBT Grants; Includes New States, Rural Communities*, June 28, 2017, https://www.fns.usda.gov/pressrelease/2017/006617.

[48] Ibid.

states that have not participated before, statewide projects, and projects that can operate in the summers of 2019 through 2021.[49]

Table 3. Appropriations for Summer Demonstration Projects, FY2010-FY2018

Demonstration Type	Fiscal Year	Appropriation ($ in millions)
All summer demonstration projects	FY2010	85.0 (available until expended)
FY2011	n/a	
FY2012	n/a	
FY2013	n/a	
FY2014	n/a	
Summer EBT only	FY2015	16.0
FY2016	23.0	
FY2017	23.0	
FY2018	28.0	

Source: Enacted appropriations laws for FY2010-FY2018.

Notes: Appropriations for the summer demonstration projects are generally contained in the "Child Nutrition Programs" section of enacted appropriations acts. However, the FY2016 appropriations act included $7 million for these projects in a general provision (§741).

There were proposals in the 114th and 115th Congresses to expand Summer EBT. For example, the Senate committee's child nutrition reauthorization proposal in the 114th Congress (S. 3136) would have allowed a portion of SFSP's mandatory funding to cover Summer EBT and authorized up to $50 million in discretionary funding for the program. In addition, in its FY2017 budget proposal, the Obama Administration recommended expansion of Summer EBT nationwide with a phase-in over 10 years.[50] Freestanding bills in the 114th and 115th Congresses had similar objectives.[51]

---

[49] Grants.gov, *Summer Electronic Benefit Transfer for Children (Summer EBT) Grant Program: Fiscal Year 2019 Request for Applications*, USDA-FNS, October 31, 2018, https://www.grants.gov/web/grants/view-opportunity.html? oppId=310059.

[50] Details about the Obama Administration's Nationwide Summer EBT proposal are available in the FY2017 budget USDA-FNS Explanatory Notes on pp. 32-34, http://www.obpa.usda.gov/32fns2017notes.pdf.

[51] For example, see the Stop Child Summer Hunger Act of 2015 (S. 1539/H.R. 2715) in the 114th Congress and the Stop Child Summer Hunger Act of 2018 (H.R. 6516/S. 3268) in the 115th Congress.

Other Summer Demonstrations

Funding from the 2010 Agriculture Appropriations Act (Section 749(g) of P.L. 111-80) was also used for other demonstration projects. One of these, the Enhanced Summer Food Service Program (eSFSP), took place during the summers of 2010 through 2012 in eight states.[52] It included four initiatives: (1) incentives for SFSP sites to lengthen operations to 40 or more days, (2) funding to add recreational or educational activities at meal sites, (3) meal delivery for children in rural areas, and (4) food backpacks that children could take home on weekends and holidays.

Evaluations of eSFSP were published from 2011 to 2014. Summer meal participation rates rose during the demonstration periods for all four initiatives.[53] In addition, children in the meal delivery and backpack demonstrations had consistent rates of food insecurity from summer to fall (this was not measured for the other initiatives).[54] However, the results from these evaluations should be interpreted with caution due to a small sample size, the lack of a comparison group, and potential confounding factors.[55]

Another demonstration project, also operating under authority provided by the 2010 Agriculture Appropriations Act, provided exemptions from the congregate feeding requirement to SFSP and SSO outdoor meal sites experiencing excessive heat each summer since 2015 (as of the date of this chapter).[56] Exempted sites must continue to serve children in congregate settings on days when heat is not excessive, and

---

[52] USDA-FNS, "Enhanced Summer Food Service Program (eSFSP)," https://www.fns.usda.gov/ops/enhanced-summerfood-service-program-esfsp. The eSFSP pilot states were Arizona, Arkansas, Delaware, Kansas, Massachusetts, Mississippi, New York, and Ohio.

[53] Elinson et al., *Evaluation of the Summer Food Service Program Enhancement Demonstrations: 2012 Demonstration Evaluation Report*, prepared by Westat for USDA-FNS, 2014, https://fns-prod.azureedge.net/sites/default/files/ops/ esfsp2012.pdf.

[54] Elinson et al., *Evaluation of the Summer Food Service Program Enhancement Demonstrations: 2011 Demonstration Evaluation Report*, prepared by Westat for USDA-FNS, November 2012, https://fns-prod.azureedge.net/sites/default/files/eSFSP_2011 Demo_0.pdf.

[55] See chapter 6.2, "Study Strengths and Limitation," of Elinson et al., *Evaluation of the Summer Food Service Program Enhancement Demonstrations: 2012 Demonstration Evaluation Report*, prepared by Westat for USDA-FNS, 2014, https://fns-prod.azureedge.net/sites/default/files/ops/esfsp2012.pdf.

[56] USDA-FNS, "Demonstration Project for Non-Congregate Feeding for Outdoor Summer Meal Sites Experiencing Excessive Heat with Q&As," May 24, 2018, https://fns-prod.azureedge.net/sites/default/files/sfsp/SP14_SFSP04- 2018os.pdf.

provide meals in another form (e.g., a take-home form) on days of excessive heat. USDA also offers exemptions on a case-by-case basis for other extreme weather conditions. This demonstration has not been evaluated.

Other Proposals

There were other proposals and hearings related to congregate feeding in SFSP in recent years.[57] For example, in the 114th Congress, committee-reported child nutrition reauthorization proposals in the Senate and the House (S. 3136 and H.R. 5003, respectively) would have enabled some rural meal sites to provide SFSP meals for consumption offsite. Specifically, both proposals would have allowed offsite consumption for children (1) in rural areas (H.R. 5003 to a more limited extent than S. 3136) and (2) in nonrural areas in which more than 80% of students are certified as eligible for free or reduced-price meals. The bills would have also permitted congregate feeding sites to provide meals to be consumed offsite episodically under certain conditions such as extreme weather or public safety concerns.

Community Eligibility Provision

The HHFKA created the Community Eligibility Provision (CEP), an option to provide free meals (lunches and breakfasts) to all students in schools with high proportions of students who automatically qualify for free or reduced-price lunches.[58] CEP became available to schools

---

[57] For example, see S. 613/H.R. 1728 and S. 1966 in the 114th Congress and H.R. 203 in the 115th Congress. During 114th Congress hearings, witnesses testified about SFSP and summer alternatives before the House Committee on Education and the Workforce (April 15, 2015; June 16, 2015; June 24, 2015) and the Senate Committee on Agriculture, Nutrition, and Forestry (May 7, 2015). In the 115th Congress, witnesses testified about SFSP and summer alternatives before the House Subcommittee on Early Childhood, Elementary, and Secondary Education (July 17, 2018).

[58] Section 104 of the HHFKA added paragraph (F), "Universal Meal Service in High Poverty Areas" to Section 11(a)(1) of the Richard B. Russell National School Lunch Act (NSLA; 42 U.S.C. 1759a(a)(1)(F)). For more information about how CEP works, see CRS Report R43783, *School Meals Programs and Other USDA Child Nutrition Programs: A Primer.*

nationwide starting in SY2014-2015, and participation has increased since then. As of SY2016- 2017, more than 20,700 schools participated in CEP, according to data from the Food Research and Action Center (FRAC), a nonprofit advocacy organization.[59] This is roughly 22% of NSLP schools.[60]

Several groups have expressed support for CEP during its implementation, arguing that the provision improves access to meals, reduces stigma associated with receiving free or reduced-price meals, and reduces schools' administrative costs.[61] Others have sought to change the option. For example, in the 114th Congress, the House's committee-reported child nutrition reauthorization bill (H.R. 5003) would have restricted schools' eligibility for CEP, which the committee majority argued was "to better target resources to those students in need, while also ensuring all students who are eligible for assistance continue to receive assistance."[62]

Aside from CEP, schools may also provide universal free meal service through the "Provision 2" and "Provision 3" options. CEP is unique in that no school meal applications are required. For information on other options, see the USDA-FNS website, http://www.fns.usda.gov/school-meals/provisions-1-2-and-3.

[59] Food Research and Action Center, "Community Eligibility Continues to Grow in the 2016–2017 School Year," March 2017, http://www.frac.org/wp-content/uploads/CEP-Report_Final_Links_032317.pdf.

[60] The 22% represents 20,721 schools participating in CEP in SY2016-2017 out of 95,642 schools participating in NSLP in FY2017, according to participation data from USDA-FNS. This is an estimate because the time periods do not match precisely.

[61] For example, see No Kid Hungry, *How the Community Eligibility Provision (CEP) Can Help,* http://bestpractices.nokidhungry.org/programs/school-breakfast/about-the-community-eligibility-provision; Food Research and Action Center, *Facts: Community Eligibility Provision,* http://frac.org/wp-content/uploads/frac-factscommunity-eligibility-provision.pdf; and Center on Budget and Policy Priorities (CBPP), *Community Eligibility: Making High-Poverty Schools Hunger Free*, October 1, 2013, https://www.cbpp.org/research/community-eligibilitymaking-high-poverty-schools-hunger-free.

[62] U.S. Congress, House Committee on Education and the Workforce, *Improving Child Nutrition and Education Act of 2016*, report to accompany H.R. 5003, 114th Congress, 2nd session, H.Rept. 114-852, (Washington, DC: GPO, 2016), p. 54, https://www.congress.gov/114/crpt/hrpt852/CRPT-114hrpt852-pt1.pdf. Eligibility for CEP depends on a school's identified student percentage (ISP), the share of enrolled students who are identified as eligible for free school meals through direct certification. Under current law, a school, school district, or group of schools within a district must have an ISP of 40% or greater to use CEP. The House committee-reported bill would have increased this proportion to 60% or greater, reducing schools' eligibility for the option.

One secondary effect of CEP is that it has created data issues for other nonnutrition federal and state programs.[63] Many programs, most notably the federal Title I-A program (the primary source of federal funding for elementary and secondary schools), use free and reduced-price lunch data to determine eligibility and/or funding allocations. These data come from school meal applications, which are no longer collected under CEP's automatic eligibility determination process.[64]

Unpaid Meal Costs and "Lunch Shaming"

Students may qualify for free meals, or they may have to pay for reduced-price or full-price meals.[65] In recent years, the issue of students owing and not paying their meal costs, and schools' responses to such situations, has received increased attention. In many cases, schools serve students a regular meal, charging the unpaid meal cost and creating a debt that they may try to collect later from the family. In other cases, schools respond with what some have called "lunch shaming" practices—most commonly, taking or throwing away a student's selected hot foods and providing an alternative cold meal or, less commonly, barring children from participation in school events until debt is repaid or having children wear a visual indicator of meal debt (e.g., a stamp or sticker). Lunch shaming instances have largely been reported in news articles from different states, and there are limited national data available on the

---

[63] Ibid, p. 163.

[64] Also see M. Levin and Z. Neuberger, *Improving Direct Certification Will Help More Low-Income Children Receive School Meals*, Center on Budget and Policy Priorities, and Food Research and Action Center, July 25, 2014, p. 3, https://www.cbpp.org/researc h/food-assistance/implications-of-community-eligibility-for-the-education-ofdisadvantaged.

[65] Exceptions include Community Eligibility Provision (CEP) schools/districts, which provide free meals to all students. Some have noted that providing free meals to all students can prevent lunch shaming. See, for example, James Weill, "How to stop school lunch shaming? Leave kids out of it," *The Hill*, http://thehill.com/blogs/pundits-blog/ education/333003-how-to-stop-school-lunch-shaming-leave-kids-out-of-it; U.S. Department of Agriculture, *Report to Congress: Review of Local Policies on Meal Charges and Provision of Alternate Meals*, June 2016, at https://fnsprod.azureedge.net/sites/default/ files/cn/unpaidmealcharges-report.pdf.

prevalence of such practices (available data are discussed in the text box below).[66]

Many school districts report that unpaid meal costs create a financial burden on their meal programs (see text box below for more detail).[67] In addition to federal funds, student payments for full and reduced-price meals are a primary source of revenue for school food programs. Schools have an interest in collecting this revenue to help fund operations.[68] Also, according to federal regulations, if schools are unable to recover unpaid meal funds, the money becomes "bad debt" and the school or school district must use other nonfederal funding sources to cover the costs.[69]

Starting in 2010, Congress and USDA have taken actions to address the issue of unpaid meal costs. Section 143 of the HHFKA required USDA to examine states' and school districts' policies and practices regarding unpaid meal charges. As part of the review, the law required USDA to "prepare a report on the feasibility of establishing national standards for meal charges and the provision of alternate meals" and, if applicable, make recommendations related to the implementation of the standards. The law also permitted USDA to take follow-up actions based on the findings from the report.[70]

---

[66] See, for example, B. Duhart, *Kids banned from field day if they owe lunch money. School says there's a $55,000 tab*, NJ.com, June 13, 2018, https://www.nj.com/camden/index.ssf/2018/06/ parent_claims_district_lunch_shams_kids_officials.html; S. Brown, *Mass. Bill To Prevent 'Meal Shaming' Of Schoolchildren Unlikely To Pass This Session*, WBUR.org, May 15, 2018, http://www.wbur.org/edify/2018/05/15/ meal-shaming-bill; I. Hrynkiw, *'I need lunch money,' Alabama school stamps on child's arm*, AL.com, June 13, 2016, https://www.al.com/news/birmingham/index.ssf/2016/06/gardendale_elementary_student.html; Dallas Morning News, *Texas children could use school food pantry, avoid lunch shaming under proposed legislation*, April 20, 2017, https://www.dallasnews.com/news/education/2017/04/20/texas-children-use-school-food-pantry-avoid-lunch-shamingproposed-legislation.

[67] USDA, *Report to Congress: Review of Local Policies on Meal Charges and Provision of Alternate Meals*, June 2016, p. 5, https://fns-prod.azureedge.net/sites/default/files/cn/unpaidmealcharges-report.pdf.

[68] USDA-FNS, "Unpaid Meal Charges: Clarification on Collection of Delinquent Meal Payments," July 8, 2016, p. 2, https://fns-prod.azureedge.net/sites/default/files/cn/SP47-2016os.pdf.

[69] 7 C.F.R. 200.426.

[70] Specifically, Section 143 of the HHFKA authorized USDA to (1) implement standards, (2) implement demonstration projects, or (3) further study the feasibility of the recommendations.

USDA's subsequent Report to Congress in June 2016 ultimately did *not* recommend national standards, but instead recommended "clarifying and updating policy guidance on specific national policies impacting unpaid meal charges and facilitating the development and distribution of best practices to support decision making by States and localities."[71] USDA-FNS followed up with a memorandum requiring SFAs to institute and communicate, by July 1, 2017, a written meal charge policy, which was to include instructions on how to address situations in which a child does not pay for a meal.[72] USDA-FNS also provided clarification through webinars, other memoranda, and a best practice guide.[73]

In the Report to Congress, USDA stated that its recommendation was based on findings from a study published by USDA-FNS in March 2014 and a Request for Information (RFI) on "Unpaid Meal Charges" published by USDA-FNS in October 2014.[74] The findings from both the study and the RFI—which garnered 462 comments—showed that meal charge policies were largely determined at the school and school district levels rather than the state level. The responses to the RFI also indicated that such policies ranged in formality, with varying degrees of review (e.g., some required school board approval while others did not) and enforcement. In the RFI comments, school and district officials generally expressed a preference for local control of meal charge policies, while national advocacy groups generally favored national standards.

---

[71] USDA, *Report to Congress: Review of Local Policies on Meal Charges and Provision of Alternate Meals*, June 2016, p. 5, https://fns-prod.azureedge.net/sites/default/files/cn/unpaidmealcharges-report.pdf.

[72] USDA-FNS, "Unpaid Meal Charges: Local Meal Charge Policies," July 8, 2016, https://fns-prod.azureedge.net/sites/ default/files/cn/SP46-2016os.pdf. The best practice guide is called "2017 Edition: Overcoming the Unpaid Meal Challenge: Proven Strategies from Our Nation's Schools," available at https://www.fns.usda.gov/school-meals/2017- edition-overcoming-unpaid-meal-challenge-proven-strategies-our-nations-schools.

[73] For a list of resources, see USDA-FNS, "Unpaid Meal Charges," https://www.fns.usda.gov/school-meals/unpaidmeal-charges.

[74] May et al., Special Nutrition Program Operations Study: State and School Food Authority Policies and Practices for School Meals Programs School Year 2011-12, prepared by Westat under Contract No. AG-3198-D-10-0048 (Alexandria, VA: USDA-FNS, March 2014), pp. 147-148, https://fns-prod.azureedge.net/sites/default/files/ SNOPSYear1.pdf; USDA-FNS, "Request for Information: Unpaid Meal Charges," 79 Federal Register 62095, October 16, 2014, https://www.regulations.gov/docketBrowser?rpp=25&po=0&dct=PS&D=FNS-2014-0039.

Data on Unpaid Meal Costs and "Lunch Shaming"

There are limited national data available on the prevalence of "lunch shaming" practices. However, there are data on unpaid meal costs and schools' reported responses to these costs. For example, USDA-FNS's study published in March 2014 examined the policies and practices of a nationally representative sample of SFAs in SY2011-2012. That study found that 58% of SFAs reported incurring unpaid meal charges prior to recovery attempts.[75] Of these SFAs, 50.4% served the equivalent of a reimbursable meal to students unable to pay, 38.0% served an alternative meal (e.g., a cold meal), 5.4% combined these approaches, 4.9% did something else, and 1.3% did not serve a meal.[76] On average, SFAs recovered 31% of lost revenues from unpaid meals.

USDA-FNS's RFI published in October 2014 also shed light on schools' and school districts' perspectives and policies regarding unpaid meal charges.[77] According to USDA's analysis of the comments, many school and district officials said that they allowed a certain number of charges before providing an alternative meal or cutting students off from meals.[78] The most common reported alternative meal was a cheese or peanut butter and jelly sandwich, a fruit or vegetable, and unflavored milk. Generally, school districts' policies were more lenient for elementary school students and stricter for middle and high school students. Many officials reported that unpaid meal charges were a financial burden on their school food service account, both in terms of lost revenue and the costs associated with collecting debt from families.

The topics of lunch shaming and unpaid meal costs also surfaced in the 115th Congress. For example, a provision in the FY2018 appropriations law stated that funds appropriated in the law could not be used in ways that result in discrimination against children eligible for free or reduced-price meals, including the practices of segregating children and overtly identifying children by special tokens or tickets (note that this does not

---

[75] May et al., *Special Nutrition Program Operations Study: State and School Food Authority Policies and Practices for School Meals Programs School Year 2011-12*, prepared by Westat under Contract No. AG-3198-D-10-0048 (Alexandria, VA: USDA-FNS, March 2014), pp. 147-148, https://fns-prod.azureedge.net/sites/default/files/ SNOPSYear1.pdf.

[76] Ibid.

[77] USDA-FNS, "Request for Information: Unpaid Meal Charges," 79 *Federal Register* 62095, October 16, 2014, https://www.regulations.gov/docketBrowser?rpp=25&po=0&dct=PS&D=FNS-2014-0039.

[78] USDA, *Report to Congress: Review of Local Policies on Meal Charges and Provision of Alternate Meals*, June 2016, p. 3-5, https://fns-prod.azureedge.net/sites/default/files/cn/unpaidmealcharges-report.pdf.

pertain to children paying for full-price meals).[79] Legislative proposals in the 115th Congress included the Anti-Lunch Shaming Act of 2017 (H.R. 2401/S. 1064), which sought to establish national standards for how schools treat children unable to pay for a meal.[80]

Unpaid meal costs and lunch shaming have also been active topics at the state level. In recent years, a number of states have enacted legislation aimed at addressing these issues.[81] For example, in 2018, Illinois passed legislation that requires schools to serve a regular (reimbursable) meal to students who do not pay and allows school districts to request an offset from the state for debts exceeding $500.[82]

Paid Lunch and Other School Food Pricing

The HHFKA created new requirements related to schools' pricing of paid lunches (sometimes referred to as "paid lunch equity" requirements).[83] Specifically, the law required all NSLP participating SFAs to review their average price of paid lunches and, if necessary, gradually increase prices based on a formula.[84] The law also gave SFAs the option to meet the

---

[79] See Section 768 (Title VII of Division A) of P.L. 115-141, which references Section 9(b)(10) of the Richard B. Russell National School Lunch Act (42 U.S.C. 1758(b)(10)) and 7 C.F.R. 245.8.

[80] Specifically, the legislation would have prohibited SFAs from (1) publicly identifying children who cannot pay for a meal or those who have meal debt, (2) having those children perform chores or other activities, and (3) throwing away a child's meal. See Section 2 of H.R. 2401 and S. 1064 (identical text).

[81] School Nutrition Association, *State Legislation and Policy Reports*, 2016-2018, https://schoolnutrition.org/ uploadedFiles/Legislation_and_Policy/State_and_Local_Legislation_and_Regulations/SNA -2018-Third-Quarter-StateLegislative-Report.pdf; D. Temkin, and A. Cox, *State policies to address school lunch shaming*, Child Trends, February 2018, https://www.childtrends.org/ state-policies-address-school-lunch-shaming.

[82] Illinois State Legislature, Hunger-Free Students' Bill of Rights Act (Public Act 100-1092), https://legiscan.com/IL/ bill/SB2428/2017.

[83] Section 205 of P.L. 111-296, codified at 42 U.S.C. 1760(p) and 7 C.F.R. 210.14.

[84] 7 C.F.R. 210.14 and Section 12(p) of the Richard B. Russell National School Lunch Act (42 U.S.C. 1760(p)).

requirements with specified nonfederal funding sources instead of raising prices.[85]

According to the Senate committee report on the HHFKA, the requirements were intended "to ensure that children receiving free and reduced price lunches receive the full value of federal funds."[86] Prior to the paid lunch equity requirements, a USDA study found that federal subsidies for free and reduced-price lunches were cross-subsidizing other aspects of the meals programs, likely including paid lunches.[87] This can occur because federal reimbursements for free, reduced-price, and paid lunches are all mixed into the same SFA-run "nonprofit school food service account" (NSFSA).[88] Some observers argue, however, that raising prices may reduce participation in paid lunches.[89]

Under the paid lunch equity formula, the price per paid lunch must eventually match or exceed the difference between the federal reimbursements for free and paid lunches. If this is not the case, schools must increase prices over time until they make up the difference. For example, the federal reimbursement was $3.37 for free lunches and $0.37 for paid lunches SY2018-2019 for some schools.[90] Under the requirements, if schools were not charging at least $3.00 per paid lunch, they would be

---

[85] Ibid. Financial support from nonfederal sources must be "for the direct support for paid lunches." Revenue from competitive foods and funds specified for the School Breakfast Program, free or reduced-price lunches, or other child nutrition programs cannot be used.

[86] U.S. Congress, Senate Committee on Agriculture, Nutrition, and Forestry, *Healthy, Hunger-Free Kids Act of 2010*, report to accompany S. 3307, 111th Congress, 2nd session, S.Rept. 111-178, (Washington, DC: GPO, 2010), pp. 37-38, https://www.congress.gov/111/crpt/srpt178/CRPT-111srpt178.pdf.

[87] S. Bartlett, F. Glantz, and C. Logan, *School Lunch and Breakfast Cost Study-II,* USDA-FNS, Office of Research, Nutrition and Analysis, final report, April 2008, https://www.fns.usda.gov/school-lunch-and-breakfast-cost-study-ii.

[88] 7 C.F.R. 210.14. These three meal categories are subsidized by the federal government in increasing amounts. For example, in school year 2018-19, the federal reimbursement was $0.37 for paid lunches, $2.97 for reduced-price lunches, and $3.37 for free lunches for many schools.

[89] For example, see School Nutrition Association, *2015 Position Paper Reauthorization of the Healthy, Hunger-Free Kids Act: Modify Section 205*, https://schoolnutrition.org/uploadedFiles/Legislation_and_Policy/SNA_Policy_Resources/6-2015PP-PaidLunchEquityOnePager.pdf.

[90] USDA-FNS, "National School Lunch, Special Milk, and School Breakfast Programs, National Average Payments/Maximum Reimbursement Rates," 83 *Federal Register* 34105, July, 19, 2018, https://www.federalregister.gov/documents/2018/07/19/2018-15465/national-school-lunch-special-milk-and-schoolbreakfast-programs-national-average-paymentsmaximum.

required to increase the price of a paid lunch gradually, based on a formula, until they closed the gap (see Figure 1). Schools cannot be required to raise the price by more than 10 cents annually, but they may choose to do so.

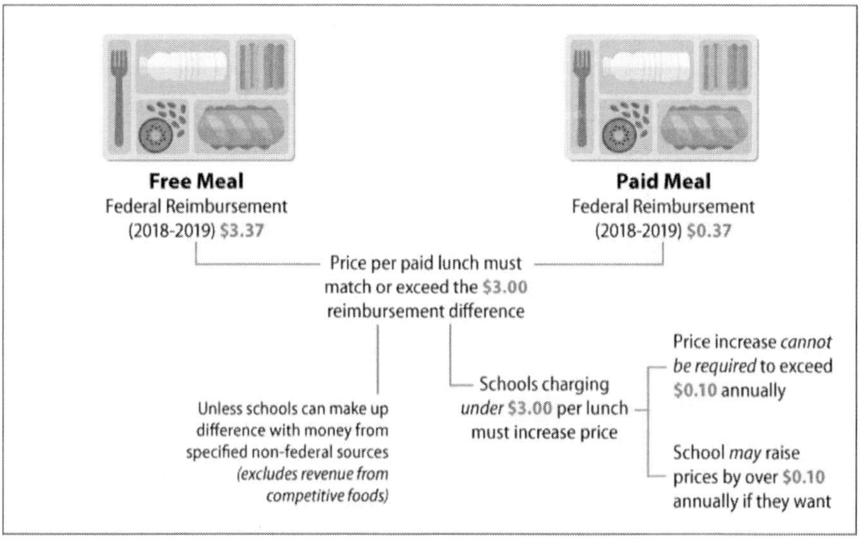

Source: CRS, based on Section 205 of P.L. 111-296.

Notes: If schools are charging under the reimbursement difference (based on their average price of a paid lunch in October of the previous school year), they must increase the price of paid lunches by at least 2% plus the percentage change in food inflation. Schools may round down to the nearest $0.05.

Figure 1. Paid Lunch Equity Formula. An Example of Schools' Pricing of Paid Lunches under the Healthy, Hunger-Free Kids Act of 2010 Using SY2018-2019 Reimbursement Rates.

The HHFKA also included related requirements for revenue from "nonprogram" (i.e., competitive) foods.[91] The law required that any revenue from nonprogram foods accrue to the SFA-run NSFSA. In practice, this prevents revenue from competitive foods from being used for other school purposes outside of food service. The law also required that, broadly speaking, revenue from nonprogram foods equal or exceed the

[91] Section 206 of P.L. 111-296.

costs of obtaining nonprogram foods (see the regulations for a specific formula).[92]

In June 2011, USDA-FNS published an interim final rule implementing the requirements starting in SY2011-2012, offering some flexibility for that first year.[93] USDA subsequently provided certain exemptions through agency guidance for SY2013-2014 through SY2017-2018 for SFAs "in strong financial standing," as determined by state agencies based on different criteria.[94] For SY2018-2019, the enacted FY2018 appropriation (Section 775 of P.L. 115-141) expanded the exemptions, requiring only SFAs with a negative balance in the NSFSA as of January 31, 2018, potentially to have to raise prices for paid meals.[95]

Other legislative proposals related to the paid lunch equity requirements were considered in recent Congresses. For example, the House committee's child nutrition reauthorization proposal in the 114th Congress would have eliminated the requirements.[96] The Senate committee's proposal would have replaced the requirements with a broader "non-federal revenue target," which could have come from household payments for full-price lunches or other state and local contributions.[97]

---

[92] 7 C.F.R. 210.14.

[93] USDA-FNS, "National School Lunch Program: School Food Service Account Revenue Amendments Related to the Healthy, Hunger-Free Kids Act of 2010," 76 *Federal Register* 35301, June 17, 2011, https://www.federalregister.gov/ documents/2011/06/17/2011-14926/national-school-lunch-program-school-food-service-account-revenue-amendments-related-to-the-healthy.

[94] USDA-FNS, *Paid Lunch Equity: Guidance for School Years 2015-16 and 2016 -2017*, February 9, 2015, https://www.fns.usda.gov/paid-lunch-equity-guidance-sys-2015-16-and-2016-17; and USDA-FNS, *Paid Lunch Equity: Guidance for School Year 2017-18,* January 12, 2017, https://fns-prod.azureedge.net/sites/default/files/cn/SP17- 2017os.pdf. Criteria included whether the SFA had been certified as meeting the meal pattern requirements, if the SFA was taking steps toward meeting the competitive foods standards, and if the increase would cause the SFA to exceed a balance limit on the nonprofit school food service account.

[95] Also see USDA-FNS, "Paid Lunch Equity: Guidance for School Year 2018-19," April 19, 2018, https://fnsprod.azureedge.net/sites/default/files/cn/SP12-2018os.pdf.

[96] Section 105(e) of H.R. 5003.

[97] Section 106 of S. 3136.

APPENDIX. ACRONYMS USED IN THIS CHAPTER

CACFP	Child and Adult Care Food Program
CDF	Canned, dried, or frozen
CEP	Community Eligibility Provision
eSFSP	Enhanced Summer Food Service Program
FFVP	Fresh Fruit and Vegetable Program
HHFKA	Healthy, Hunger-Free Kids Act
NSFSA	Nonprofit school food service account
NSLP	National School Lunch Program
SBP	School Breakfast Program
SFA	School food authority
SFSP	Summer Food Service Program
SMP	Special Milk Program
SSO	Summer Seamless Option
Summer EBT or SEBTC	Summer Electronic Benefit Transfer for Children
SY	school year
USDA-FNS	U.S. Department of Agriculture Food and Nutrition Service

In: Child Nutrition Programs
Editor: Daniel D. Coleman
ISBN: 978-1-53615-764-2

Chapter 2

An Introduction to Child Nutrition Reauthorization*

Kara Clifford Billings and Randy Alison Aussenberg

The child nutrition programs and the Special Supplemental Nutrition Program for Women, Infants, and Children (WIC) were last reauthorized in 2010. Some of the authorities created or extended in that law (Healthy, Hunger-Free Kids Act of 2010, P.L. 111-296) expired on September 30, 2015. However, the vast majority of program operations have continued with funding provided by appropriations acts.

Child nutrition reauthorization refers to Congress's process of making changes, additions, and deletions to the permanent statutes that authorize the child nutrition programs, WIC, and related policies: (1) Richard B. Russell National School Lunch Act, (2) Child Nutrition Act, and sometimes (3) Section 32 of the Act of August 24, 1935.

---

* This is an edited, reformatted and augmented version of Congressional Research Service Publication No. IF10266, updated March 8, 2019.

During the 114th Congress, committees of jurisdiction marked up bills but reauthorization was not completed (see CRS Report R44373, Tracking the Next Child Nutrition Reauthorization: An Overview).

MAJOR PROGRAMS TYPICALLY AMENDED IN A CHILD NUTRITION REAUTHORIZATION

Table 1 summarizes the major programs that have been part of a child nutrition reauthorization. There are smaller grant programs or school meals' support functions that are not listed. The five main child nutrition programs are the

- National School Lunch Program (NSLP);
- School Breakfast Program (SBP);
- Child and Adult Care Food Program (CACFP);
- Summer Food Service Program (SFSP); and
- Special Milk Program (SMP).

Participating children (and adults for CACFP) receive subsidized meals, snacks and/or milk, which may be free or at reduced price for those eligible. States and food-serving institutions (e.g., schools) receive federal reimbursements for the food served. Some programs also receive USDA commodity food assistance. Details vary by program.

WIC provides eligible low-income women, infants, and children (under five years old) with specific supplemental foods as well as certain services. The *WIC Farmers Market Nutrition Program (FMNP)* provides vouchers redeemable at farmers markets to WIC participants.

Related Programs and Policies in the Farm Bill

The Fresh Fruit and Vegetable ("Snack") Program (FFVP) is authorized in the Richard B. Russell National School Lunch Act. Omnibus farm bill legislation in 2008 and 2014 amended the program. No amendments to FFVP were made in the 2010 child nutrition reauthorization or the 2018 farm bill. The 2018 farm bill (P.L. 115-334) reauthorized the Supplemental Nutrition Assistance Program (SNAP) as well as USDA's purchase of foods for the child nutrition programs.

Categorization of Programs' Funding

Most of the WIC and child nutrition programs' funding requires annual appropriations:

- Most child nutrition program funding is appropriated mandatory spending based on formulas and criteria in the authorizing laws (e.g., the programs' per-meal reimbursements).
- Some smaller child nutrition grants and activities are funded with discretionary appropriations (e.g., Team Nutrition).
- WIC and WIC FMNP funds are discretionary.

The child nutrition programs also receive support from sources outside the appropriations process. Particularly, USDA's Section 32 program, a permanent appropriation of 30% of the previous year's customs receipts, transfers certain funds to the child nutrition programs annually.

Last Reauthorization

The 2010 reauthorization, the Healthy, Hunger-Free Kids Act of 2010 (P.L. 111-296), included a number of new and revised policies, particularly for the school meals programs (NSLP and SBP). In some cases, the new policies' details are largely described within the statute (e.g., community eligibility provision, an option for eligible schools to provide all meals for free). In other cases, the details of the policy were laid out in USDA-promulgated regulations (e.g., updated school meals nutrition standards and new nutrition standards for other foods sold in schools).

Have the Programs Expired?

Many of these programs' authorizations are permanent (they have no expiration date). This is the case for the main functions of NSLP, SBP, CACFP, and SMP.

In other cases, while the authority for the program itself is permanent, the program's authorization of appropriations expired on September 30, 2015 (e.g., SFSP, WIC, WIC FMNP, and State Administrative Expenses, which funds states' operation of certain programs). In such cases, the program may still operate if funding is provided in appropriations laws, which has been the case for these programs in FY2016 (P.L. 114-113), FY2017 (P.L. 115- 31), FY2018 (P.L. 115-141), and FY2019 (P.L. 116-6) (as well as FY2016, FY2017, FY2018, and FY2019 continuing resolutions).

A few pilot programs and temporary activities expired on September 30, 2015, and were not always extended. A California program to provide SFSP snacks year-round has not been extended. Currently, federal authority to conduct food safety audits and mandatory funding for a National Hunger Clearinghouse have been extended by FY2017, FY2018, and FY2019 appropriations laws.

Table 1. Child Nutrition and WIC Programs at a Glance

Program	Authorizing Statute (Year First Authorized)	Distinguishing Characteristics	FY2018 Expenditures (exceptions noted)	FY2018 Average Daily Participation (exceptions noted)
National School Lunch	Richard B. Russell	Lunches at school	$13.8 billion	29.7 million
Program	National School Lunch Act	Typically served in schools, to pre-K-12		
	(1946)	students, during the school day and year Possible to provide summer food and afterschool snacks		
School Breakfast Program	Child Nutrition Act (1966)	Breakfasts at school (also for pre-K-12) Typically served in schools, to K-12 students, during the school day and year	$4.4 billion	14.7 million
Child and Adult Care	Richard B. Russell	Meals and snacks in early childhood and adult	$3.6 billion	4.5 million
Food Program (child care center, day care homes, adult day care centers)	National School Lunch Act (1968)	day care settings Rules and funding differ based on type of institution	(includes at-risk after-school spending, described below)	children; 131,700 adults
Child and Adult Care	Richard B. Russell	Supper and snacks for school-age children	(not available;	1.9 million
Food Program (at-risk after-school snacks and meals)[a]	National School Lunch Act (1994)	after-school	included in CACFP total above)	children (included in CACFP children above)
Summer Food Service Program	Richard B. Russell National School Lunch Act (1968)	Meals and snacks provided during summer months Sites vary and include schools, community centers, camps, parks, and others Eligibility rules vary by type of site	$472 million	145.8 million meals served annually[b]

Table 1. (Continued)

Program	Authorizing Statute (Year First Authorized)	Distinguishing Characteristics	FY2018 Expenditures (exceptions noted)	FY2018 Average Daily Participation (exceptions noted)
Special Milk Program	Child Nutrition Act (1954)	Subsidizes milk, not meals or snacks Institutions eligible must not participate in NSLP or SBP	$7.9 million	37.9 million half-pints average monthly
Special Supplemental Nutrition Program for Women, Infants, and Children (WIC)	Child Nutrition Act (1974)	Provides benefits redeemable for supplemental foods; and nutrition counseling, and breastfeeding support, to pregnant, breastfeeding, and postpartum women; infants; and children (under five years old).	$6.1 billion (FY2019 appropriations)[c]	6.9 million average Monthly (preliminary FY2018 data)
WIC Farmers' Market Nutrition Program (WIC FMNP)	Child Nutrition Act (1992)	Provides vouchers for WIC participants to redeem at farmers' markets.	$18.5 million (FY2019 appropriations)	1.7 million recipients total in FY2017
Fresh Fruit and Vegetable Program (FFVP)	Richard B. Russell National School Lunch Act (2002)	Provides free fresh fruit and vegetable snacks to elementary school students	$167.5 million (transfer from Section 32)[d]	Not available

Source: Except as noted, participation and funding data from USDA-FNS Key Data Report, January 2019, based on data through November 2018. WIC, WIC FMNP FY2018 appropriations from P.L. 115-141 and related documents.

[a] At-risk after-school snacks and meals are part of CACFP law and funding, but differ in their rules and the age of children served.

[b] In a May 2018 report, GAO found that average daily participation estimates in SFSP were unreliable (for more information, see GAO, Actions Needed to Improve Participation Estimates and Address Program Challenges, GAO-18-369, May 31, 2018).

[c] Section 723 of P.L. 116-5 also rescinded $500 million in prior-year carryover funding.

[d] FY2018 allocation, not expenditures. USDA-FNS policy memorandum SP 35-2017, FFVP FY2018 Funding Allocation, June 2017.

In: Child Nutrition Programs
Editor: Daniel D. Coleman ISBN: 978-1-53615-764-2

Chapter 3

SCHOOL MEALS PROGRAMS AND OTHER USDA CHILD NUTRITION PROGRAMS: A PRIMER (UPDATED)*

Kara Clifford Billings and Randy Alison Aussenberg

ABSTRACT

The "child nutrition programs" refer to the U.S. Department of Agriculture's Food and Nutrition Service (USDA-FNS) programs that provide food for children in school or institutional settings. The best known programs, which serve the largest number of children, are the school meals programs: the National School Lunch Program (NSLP) and the School Breakfast Program (SBP). The child nutrition programs also include the Child and Adult Care Food Program (CACFP), which provides meals and snacks in day care and after school settings; the Summer Food Service Program (SFSP), which provides food during the summer months; the Special Milk Program (SMP), which supports milk for schools that do not participate in NSLP or SBP; and the Fresh Fruit

---

* This is an edited, reformatted and augmented version of Congressional Research Service, Publication No. R43783, dated February 11, 2019.

and Vegetable Program (FFVP), which funds fruit and vegetable snacks in select elementary schools.

Funding: The vast majority of the child nutrition programs account is considered mandatory spending, with trace amounts of discretionary funding for certain related activities. Referred to as open-ended, "appropriated entitlements," funding is provided through the annual appropriations process; however, the level of *spending* is controlled by benefit and eligibility criteria in federal law and dependent on the resulting levels of participation. Federal cash funding (in the form of per-meal reimbursements) and USDA commodity food support is guaranteed to schools and other providers based on the number of meals or snacks served and participant category (e.g., free meals for poor children get higher subsidies).

Participation: The child nutrition programs serve children of varying ages and in different institutional settings. The NSLP and SBP have the broadest reach, serving qualifying children of all ages in school settings. Other child nutrition programs serve more-narrow populations. CACFP, for example, provides meals and snacks to children in early childhood and after-school settings among other venues. Programs generally provide some subsidy for all food served but a larger federal reimbursement for food served to children from low-income households.

Administration: Responsibility for child nutrition programs is divided between the federal government, states, and localities. The state agency and type of local provider differs by program. In the NSLP and SBP, schools and school districts ("school food authorities") administer the program. Meanwhile, SFSP (and sometimes CACFP) uses a model in which sponsor organizations handle administrative responsibilities for a number of sites that serve meals.

Reauthorization: The underlying laws covering the child nutrition programs were last reauthorized in the Healthy, Hunger-Free Kids Act of 2010 (HHFKA, P.L. 111-296, enacted December 13, 2010). This law made significant changes to child nutrition programs, including increasing federal financing for school lunches, expanding access to community eligibility and direct certification options for schools, and expanding eligibility options for home child care providers. The law also required an update to school meal nutrition guidelines as well as new guidelines for food served outside the meal programs (e.g., snacks sold in vending machines and cafeteria a la carte lines).

Current Issues: The 114th Congress began but did not complete a 2016 child nutrition reauthorization, and there was no significant legislative activity with regard to reauthorization in the 115th Congress. However, the vast majority of operations and activities continue with funding provided by appropriations laws.

INTRODUCTION AND BACKGROUND

The federal child nutrition programs provide assistance to schools and other institutions in the form of cash, commodity food, and administrative support (such as technical assistance and administrative funding) based on the provision of meals and snacks to children.[1] In general, these programs were created (and amended over time) to both improve children's nutrition and provide support to the agriculture economy.

Today, the child nutrition programs refer primarily to the following meal, snack, and milk reimbursement programs (these and other acronyms are listed in Appendix A):[2]

- National School Lunch Program (NSLP) (Richard B. Russell National School Lunch Act (42 U.S.C. 1751 et seq.));
- School Breakfast Program (SBP) (Child Nutrition Act, Section 4 (42 U.S.C. 1773));
- Child and Adult Care Food Program (CACFP) (Richard B. Russell National School Lunch Act, Section 17 (42 U.S.C. 1766));
- Summer Food Service Program (SFSP) (Richard B. Russell National School Lunch Act, Section 13 (42 U.S.C. 1761)); and
- Special Milk Program (SMP) (Child Nutrition Act, Section 3 (42 U.S.C. 1772)).

The programs provide financial support and/or foods to the institutions that prepare meals and snacks served outside of the home (unlike other food assistance programs such as the Supplemental Nutrition Assistance

---

[1] As discussed later in the report, the Child and Adult Care Food Program (CACFP) also supports food in adult day care facilities, but the child nutrition programs overwhelmingly serve children.

[2] Some lists also include the Fresh Fruit and Vegetable Program (FFVP) (Richard B. Russell National School Lunch Act, Section 19 (42 U.S.C. 1769a)), a newer program that is financed in a much different way than the programs listed. FFVP is discussed further later in the report ("Fresh Fruit and Vegetable Program"). WIC (the Special Supplemental Nutrition Program for Women, Infants, and Children) is also typically reauthorized with the child nutrition programs. WIC is not one of the child nutrition programs and is not discussed in this chapter.

Program (SNAP, formerly the Food Stamp Program) where benefits are used to purchase food for home consumption). Though exact eligibility rules and pricing vary by program, in general the amount of federal reimbursement is greater for meals served to qualifying low-income individuals or at qualifying institutions, although most programs provide some subsidy for all food served. Participating children receive subsidized meals and snacks, which may be free or at reduced price. Forthcoming sections discuss how program-specific eligibility rules and funding operate.

This chapter describes how each program operates under current law, focusing on eligibility rules, participation, and funding. This introductory section describes some of the background and principles that generally apply to all of the programs; subsequent sections go into further detail on the workings of each.

Unless stated otherwise, participation and funding data come from USDA-FNS's "Keydata Reports."[3]

Authorization and Reauthorization

The child nutrition programs are most often dated back to the 1946 enactment of the National School Lunch Act, which created the National School Lunch Program, albeit in a different form than it operates today.[4] Most of the child nutrition programs do *not* date back to 1946; they were added and amended in the decades to follow as policymakers expanded child nutrition programs' institutional settings and meals provided:

---

[3] This CRS report uses the May 2018 report, which contains data through March 2018. Keydata Reports available at http://www.fns.usda.gov/data-and-statistics.

[4] P.L. 79-396. There were, however, a number of smaller, more temporary precursor school food programs prior to 1946; see Gordon W. Gunderson, *National School Lunch Program: Background and Development*, 1971, http://www.fns.usda.gov/nslp/history. The 1946 law supported school lunch programs by giving formula grant funding to states based on factors such as per capita income, rather than the current-day open-ended entitlements based largely on eligibility and participation rules.

- The Special Milk Program was created in 1954, regularly extended, and made permanent in 1970.[5]
- The School Breakfast Program was piloted in 1966, regularly extended, and eventually made permanent in 1975.[6]
- A program for child care settings and summer programs was piloted in 1968, with separate programs authorized in 1975 and then made permanent in 1978.[7] These are now the Child and Adult Care Food Program[8] and Summer Food Service Program.
- The Fresh Fruit and Vegetable Program began as a pilot in 2002, was made permanent in 2004, and was expanded nationwide in 2008.[9]

The programs are now authorized under three major federal statutes: the Richard B. Russell National School Lunch Act (originally enacted as the National School Lunch Act in 1946), the Child Nutrition Act (originally enacted in 1966), and Section 32 of the act of August 24, 1935 (7 U.S.C. 612c).[10] Congressional jurisdiction over the underlying three laws has typically been exercised by the Senate Agriculture, Nutrition, and Forestry Committee; the House Education and the Workforce Committee; and, to a limited extent (relating to commodity food assistance and Section 32 issues), the House Agriculture Committee.

Congress periodically reviews and reauthorizes expiring authorities under these laws. The child nutrition programs were most recently reauthorized in 2010 through the Healthy, Hunger-Free Kids Act of 2010 (HHFKA, P.L. 111-296); some of the authorities created or extended in

---

[5] P.L. 83-690 and P.L. 91-295. Milk purchases and donations for schools did exist prior to the 1954 law.

[6] Gordon W. Gunderson, *National School Lunch Program: Background and Development*, 1971, http://www.fns.usda.gov/nslp/history.

[7] P.L. 90-302, P.L. 94-105, P.L. 95-627. Institute of Medicine, *Child and Adult Care Food Program: Aligning Dietary Guidance for All*, 2011, p. 30, https://www.nap.edu/catalog/12959/child-and-adult-care-food-program-aligning-dietaryguidance-for.

[8] Adult day care was added in 1987 (Older Americans Act Amendments of 1987; P.L. 100-175).

[9] P.L. 107-171; P.L. 108-265; P.L. 110-246.

[10] In 1999, P.L. 106-78 renamed the National School Lunch Act in Senator Richard B. Russell's honor.

that law expired on September 30, 2015.[11] WIC (the Special Supplemental Nutrition Program for Women, Infants, and Children) is also typically reauthorized with the child nutrition programs. WIC is *not* one of the child nutrition programs and is not discussed in this chapter.[12]

The 114th Congress began but did not complete a 2016 child nutrition reauthorization. There was no significant legislative activity with regard to reauthorization in the 115th Congress.

Program Administration: Federal, State, and Local

The U.S. Department of Agriculture's Food and Nutrition Service (USDA-FNS) administers the programs at the federal level. The programs are operated by a wide variety of local public and private providers and the degree of direct state involvement differs by program and state.[13] At the state level, education, health, social services, and agriculture departments all have roles; at a minimum, they are responsible for approving and overseeing local providers such as schools, summer program sponsors, and child care centers and day care homes, as well as making sure they receive the federal support they are due. At the local level, program benefits are provided to millions of children (e.g., there were 30.0 million in the National School Lunch Program, the largest of the programs, in FY2017), through some 100,000 public and private schools and residential child care institutions, nearly 170,000 child care centers and family day care homes, and just over 50,000 summer program sites.

[11] Reimbursements for NSLP, SBP, CACFP, SMP, and certain related USDA activities are permanently authorized. SFSP, WIC, and WIC Farmers Market Nutrition Program, State Administrative Expenses (discussed in "Related Programs, Initiatives, and Support Activities"), and certain related USDA activities have a September 30, 2015 expiration.

[12] See CRS Report R44115, *A Primer on WIC: The Special Supplemental Nutrition Program for Women, Infants, and Children*.

[13] In the past, the federal government (via USDA-FNS) has, for certain states, taken the place of state agencies (e.g., where a state has chosen not to operate a specific program or where there is a state prohibition on aiding private schools).

All programs are available in the 50 states and the District of Columbia. Virtually all operate in Puerto Rico, Guam, and the Virgin Islands (and, in differing versions, in the Northern Marianas and American Samoa).[14]

Funding Overview

This section summarizes the nature and extent to which the programs' funding is mandatory and discretionary, including a discussion of appropriated entitlement status. Table 3 lists child nutrition program and related expenditures.

Open-Ended, Appropriated Entitlement Funding

Most spending for child nutrition programs is provided in annual appropriations acts to fulfill the legal financial obligation established by the authorizing laws. That is, the level of spending for such programs, referred to as appropriated mandatory spending, is not controlled through the annual appropriations process, but instead is derived from the benefit and eligibility criteria specified in the authorizing laws. The appropriated mandatory funding is treated as mandatory spending. Further, if Congress does not appropriate the funds necessary to fund the program, eligible entities may have legal recourse.[15] Congress typically considers the Administration's forecast for program needs in its appropriations decisions.

---

[14] For more information on child nutrition programs in the Northern Marianas and American Samoa, see U.S. Department of the Interior, Office of Insular Affairs, Region IX Federal Regional Council, Outer Pacific Committee, *FY 2016 Report on Federal Financial Assistance to the U.S. Pacific and Caribbean Islands*, May 1, 2017, p. 10, https://www.doi.gov/sites/doi.gov/files/uploads/fy16-report-on-federal-financial-assistance-to-the-insular-areas.pdf.

[15] GAO Budget Glossary, p. 13: http://www.gao.gov/products/GAO-05-734SP.

For the majority of funding discussed in this chapter, the formula that controls the funding is not capped and fluctuates based on the reimbursement rates and the number of meals/snacks served in the programs.

Reimbursable Meals

A "reimbursable meal" (or snack in the case of some programs) is a phrase used by USDA, state, and other child nutrition policy and program operators to indicate a meal (or snack) that meets federal requirements and thereby qualifies for meal reimbursement.[16]
In general, a meal or snack that is reimbursable means that it is

- served to the correctly eligible person and/or at the eligible institution, and
- in compliance with federal nutrition requirements for the meal or snack.[17]

In the school meals programs (with some variation in other programs), the highest reimbursement is paid for meals served free to eligible children, a slightly lower reimbursement is paid for meals served at a reduced price to eligible children, and a much smaller reimbursement is also paid for meals served to children who are either ineligible for assistance or not certified. For this last group, the children pay the full price as advertised but meals are still technically subsidized.

Cash Reimbursements and Commodity Foods

In the meal service programs, such as the National School Lunch Program, School Breakfast Program, summer programs, and assistance for child care centers and day care homes, federal aid is provided in the form

[16] See, for example, definition of "reimbursement" at 7 C.F.R. 210.2.

[17] The authorizing statutes for all four of the main child nutrition programs include nutritional requirements for the meals and snacks served; these are sometimes referred to as "nutrition standards," "nutrition guidelines," or "meal patterns." In most respects, the details of the requirements are specified in USDA-FNS regulations. The nutrition guidelines differ by program, largely in consideration of the age groups fed, meals/snacks authorized, and perhaps the settings in which meals are served. See program regulations for nutritional requirements: NSLP, 7 C.F.R. 210.10; SBP, 7 C.F.R. 220.8; CACFP, 7 C.F.R. 226.20; SFSP, 7 C.F.R. 225.16.

of statutorily set subsidies (reimbursements) paid for each meal/snack served that meets federal nutrition guidelines. Although all (including full-price) meals/snacks served by participating providers are subsidized, those served free or at a reduced price to lower-income children are supported at higher rates. All federal meal/snack subsidy rates are indexed annually (each July) for inflation, as are the income eligibility thresholds for free and reduced-price meals/snacks.[18] Subsequent sections discuss how a specific program's eligibility and reimbursements work.

Most subsidies are cash payments to schools or other providers, but a smaller portion of aid is provided in the form of USDA-purchased commodity foods.[19] Laws for three child nutrition programs (NSLP, CACFP, and SFSP) require the provision of commodity foods (or in some cases allow cash in lieu of commodity foods).[20]

Meal and snack service entails nonfood costs. Federal child nutrition permeal/snack subsidies may be used to cover local providers' administrative and operating costs. However, the separate direct federal payments for administrative/operating costs ("State Administrative Expenses," discussed in the "Related Programs, Initiatives, and Support Activities" section) are limited.

Other Federal Funding

In addition to the open-ended, appropriated entitlement funds summarized above, the child nutrition programs' funding also includes certain other mandatory funding[21] and a limited amount of discretionary

---

[18] Per-meal subsidies paid to providers (e.g., schools, child care centers) are indexed annually based on the CPI-U Food Away from Home Component. For family child care homes, the annual indexing is based on the CPI-U Food at Home Component.

[19] USDA commodity foods are foods purchased by the USDA for distribution to USDA nutrition programs. These programs distribute "entitlement commodities" (an amount of USDA foods to which grantees are entitled by law) as well as "bonus commodities" (USDA food purchases based on requests from the agricultural producer community). For more information, see CRS Report R42353, *Domestic Food Assistance: Summary of Programs*.

[20] See USDA-FNS Food Distribution Division resources for more information on USDA Foods and child nutrition programs, http://www.fns.usda.gov/fdd/schoolscn-usda-foods-programs.

[21] These costs are made up of Food Safety Education, Coordinated Review, Computer Support, Training and Technical Assistance, studies, payment accuracy, and Farm to School Team. See p. 32-12 of FY2019 USDA-FNS Congressional Budget Justification, available at https://www.obpa.usda.gov/32fns2019notes.pdf.

funding. Some of the activities discussed in "Related Programs, Initiatives, and Support Activities," such as Team Nutrition, are provided for with discretionary funding.

Aside from the annually appropriated funding, the child nutrition programs are also supported by certain permanent appropriations and transfers. Notably, funding for the Fresh Fruit and Vegetable Program is funded by a transfer from USDA's Section 32 program, a permanent appropriation of 30% of the previous year's customs receipts.

State, Local, and Participant Funds

Federal subsidies do not necessarily cover the full cost of the meals and snacks offered by providers. States and localities help cover program costs, as do children's families by paying charges for nonfree or reduced-price meals/snacks. There is a nonfederal cost-sharing requirement for the school meals programs (discussed below), and some states supplement school funding through additional state per-meal reimbursements or other prescribed financing arrangements.[22]

Child Nutrition Programs at a Glance

Subsequent sections of this chapter delve into the details of how each of the child nutrition programs support the service of meals and snacks in institutional settings; first, it is useful to take a broader perspective of primary program elements. Table 1 is a top-level look at the different programs that displays distinguishing characteristics (what meals are provided, in what settings, to what ages) and recent program spending.

---

[22] The School Nutrition Association, a trade association representing school meal operators and industry, tracks state policies and funding on the organization website at https://schoolnutrition.org/LegislationPolicy/ StateLegislationPolicyReports/.

Table 1. Child Nutrition Programs at a Glance

Program	Authorizing Statute (Year First Authorized)	Distinguishing Characteristics	FY2017 Expenditures	FY2017 Average Daily Participation	Maximum Daily Snack/Meals[a]
National School Lunch Program	Richard B. Russell National School Lunch Act (1946)	• Lunches at school • Typically served in schools, to pre-K-12 students, during the school day and year • Possible to provide summer food and afterschool snacks.	$13.6 billion	30.0 million children	One meal and snack per child
School Breakfast Program	Child Nutrition Act (1966)	• Breakfasts at school (also for pre-K-12) • Typically served in schools, to pre-K-12 students, during the school day and year	$4.3 billion	14.7 million children	Generally one breakfast per child, with some flexibility
Child and Adult Care Food Program (child care centers, day care homes, adult day care centers)	Richard B. Russell National School Lunch Act (1968)	• Meals and snacks in early childhood and adult day care settings • Rules and funding differ based on type of institution	$3.5 billion (includes at risk after school spending, described below)	4.4 million children; 132,000 adults	Two meals and one snack, or one meal and two snacks per participant
Child and Adult Care Food Program (At Risk After-School snacks and meals)[b]	Richard B. Russell National School Lunch Act (1994)	• Supper and snacks for school-age children after school	(Not available; included in CACFP total above)	1.7 million children (included in CACFP children above)	One meal and one snack per child
Summer Food Service Program	Richard B. Russell National School Lunch Act (1968)	• Meals and snacks provided during summer months • Sites vary and include schools, community centers, camps, parks, and others • Eligibility rules vary for "open" and "closed" sites	$485 million	2.7 million children[c]	Lunch and breakfast or lunch and one snack per child Exception: maximum of three meals for camps or programs that serve primarily migrant children

Table 1. (Continued)

Program	Authorizing Statute (Year First Authorized)	Distinguishing Characteristics	FY2017 Expenditures	FY2017 Average Daily Participation	Maximum Daily Snack/Meals[a]
Special Milk Program	Child Nutrition Act (1954)	• Subsidizes milk, not meals or snacks • Institutions eligible must not participate in NSLP or SBP	$8 million	191,000 half pints served (average daily)[d]	Not specified
Fresh Fruit and Vegetable Program	Richard B. Russell National School Lunch Act (2002)	• Provides free fresh fruit and vegetable snacks to elementary school students	$184[e] million	Not available	Not applicable

Source: Except where noted, participation and funding data from USDA-FNS Keydata May 2018 report, which contains data through March 2018. Participation data are estimated by USDA-FNS based on meals served.

a. These maximums are provided in the authorizing law for CACFP and SFSP, but specified only in regulations (7 C.F.R. 210.10(a), 220.9(a)) for NSLP and SBP.

b. At-risk after-school snacks and meals are part of CACFP law and CACFP funding, but differ in their rules and the age of children served.

c. Based only on July 2017 participation data.

d. Data from p. 32-58 of FY2019 USDA-FNS Congressional Budget Justification.

e. Obligations data displayed on p. 32-14 of FY2019 USDA-FNS Congressional Budget Justification.

SCHOOL MEALS PROGRAMS

This section discusses the school meals programs: the National School Lunch Program (NSLP) and the School Breakfast Program (SBP). Principles and concepts common to both programs are discussed first; subsections then discuss features and data unique to the NSLP and SBP, respectively.

General Characteristics

The federal school meals programs provide federal support in the form of cash assistance and USDA commodity foods; both are provided according to statutory formulas based on the number of reimbursable meals served in schools. The subsidized meals are served by both public and private nonprofit elementary and secondary schools and residential child care institutions (RCCIs)[23] that opt to enroll and guarantee to offer free or reduced-price meals to eligible low-income children. Both cash and commodity support to participating schools are calculated based on the number and price of meals served (e.g., lunch or breakfast, free or full price), but once the aid is received by the school it is used to support the overall school meal service budget, as determined by the school. This chapter focuses on the federal reimbursements and funding, but it should be noted that some states have provided state financing through additional state-specific funding.[24]

Federal law does not require schools to participate in the school meals programs. However, some states have mandated that schools provide lunch and/or breakfast, and some of these states require that their schools do so through NSLP and/or SBP.[25] The program is open to public and private schools.

A reimbursable meal requires compliance with federal school nutrition standards, which have changed throughout the history of the program based on nutritional science and children's nutritional needs. Food items not served as a complete meal meeting nutrition standards (e.g., a la carte offerings) are not reimbursable meals, and therefore are not eligible for federal per-meal, per-snack reimbursements. Following rulemaking to implement provisions in the Healthy, Hunger-Free Kids Act of 2010 (P.L.

---

[23] This CRS report refers to "schools," but it should be understood that—for NSLP and SBP—it means both schools and RCCIs. NSLP regulations, 7 C.F.R. 210.2, define RCCIs as follows: "The term 'residential child care institutions' includes, but is not limited to: homes for the mentally, emotionally or physically impaired, and unmarried mothers and their infants; group homes; halfway houses; orphanages; temporary shelters for abused children and for runaway children; long-term care facilities for chronically ill children; and juvenile detention centers. A long-term care facility is a hospital, skilled nursing facility, intermediate care facility, or distinct part thereof, which is intended for the care of children confined for 30 days or more."

[24] See School Nutrition Association, *State School Meal Mandates and Reimbursements Report: School Year 2017 2018*, https://schoolnutrition.org/uploadedFiles/Legislation_and_Policy/State_and_Local_Legislation_and_Regulations/2017-18-State-School-Meal-Mandates-and-Reimbursements.pdf.

[25] Ibid.

111-296), USDA updated the nutrition standards for reimbursable meals in January 2012 (see "Nutrition Standards" for more information). Schools serving meals that meet the updated nutrition standards are eligible for an increased reimbursement of 6 cents per lunch.

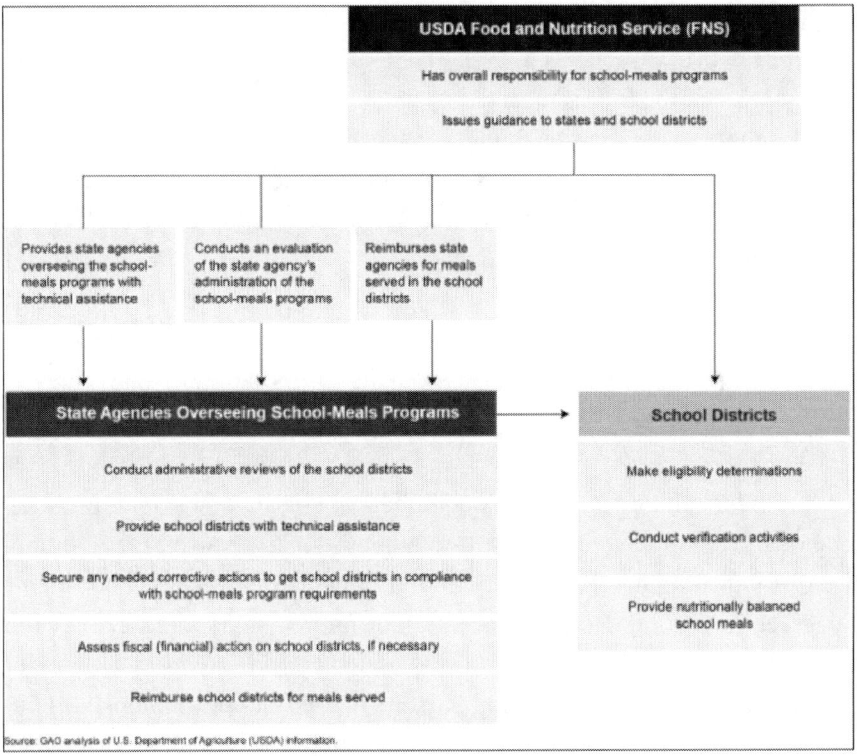

Source: Government Accountability Office (GAO), GAO-14-262, p. 47.

Figure 1. Federal, State, and Local Administration of School Meal Programs.

USDA-FNS administers the school meals programs federally, and state agencies (typically state departments of education) oversee and transmit reimbursements through agreements with school food authorities (SFAs) (typically local educational agencies (LEAs); usually these are school districts). Figure 1 provides an overview of the roles and relationships between these levels of government.

There is a cost-sharing requirement for the programs, which amounts to a contribution of approximately $200 million from the states.[26] There also are states that choose to supplement federal reimbursements with their own state reimbursements.[27]

School Meals Eligibility Rules

The school meals programs and related funding do not serve only low-income children. *All* students can receive a meal at a NSLP- or SBP-participating school, but how much the child pays for the meal and/or how much of a federal reimbursement the state receives will depend largely on whether the child qualifies for a "free," "reduced-price," or "paid" (i.e., advertised price) meal. Both NSLP and SBP use the same household income eligibility criteria and categorical eligibility rules. States and schools receive the largest reimbursements for free meals, smaller reimbursements for reduced-price meals, and the smallest (but still some federal financial support) for the full-price meals.

There are three pathways through which a child can become certified to receive a free or reduced-price meal:

1. Household income eligibility for free and reduced-price meals (information typically collected via household application),
2. Categorical (or automatic) eligibility for free meals (information collected via household application or a direct certification process), and

---

[26] Section 7(a)(1) of Richard B. Russell National School Lunch Act, codified at 42 U.S.C. 1756(a)(1). Section 7(f) of Child Nutrition Act, codified at 42 U.S.C. 1776(f).

[27] See School Nutrition Association, *State School Meal Mandates and Reimbursements Report: School Year 2017 2018*, https://schoolnutrition.org/uploadedFiles/Legislation_and_Policy/State_and_Local_Legislation_and_Regulations/2017-18-State-School-Meal-Mandates-and-Reimbursements.pdf.

3. School-wide free meals under the Community Eligibility Provision (CEP), an option for eligible schools that is based on the share of students identified as eligible for free meals.[28]

Each of these pathways is discussed in more detail below.

Income Eligibility

The income eligibility thresholds (shown in Table 2) are based on multipliers of the federal poverty guidelines. As the poverty guidelines are updated every year, so are the eligibility thresholds for NSLP and SBP.

- Free Meals: Children receive free meals if they have household income at or below 130% of the federal poverty guidelines; these meals receive the highest subsidy rate. (Reimbursements are approximately $3.30 per lunch served, less for breakfast).
- Reduced-Price Meals: Children may receive reduced-price meals (charges of no more than 40 cents for a lunch or 30 cents for a breakfast) if their household income is above 130% and less than or equal to 185% of the federal poverty guidelines; these meals receive a subsidy rate that is 40 cents (NSLP) or 30 cents (SBP) below the free meal rate. (Reimbursements are approximately $2.90 per lunch served).
- Paid Meals: A comparatively small per-meal reimbursement is provided for full-price or paid meals served to children whose families do not apply for assistance or whose family income does not qualify them for free or reduced-price meals.[29] The paid meal

[28] CEP is not the only way schools may provide universal free meal service, but it is unique in that it does not require the collection of applications.

[29] The subsidy for paid meals is provided under the authority of Section 4 of the Richard B. Russell National School Lunch Act. Section 4 establishes two different payment levels: one for schools in which *less than 60%* of the school population is participating in free or reduced-price lunch and one for schools in which *60% or more* of the school population is receiving free or reduced price lunch. See https://www.federalregister.gov/documents/2018/07/19/2018-15465/national-school-lunch-special-milk-and-school-breakfast-programs-national-average-paymentsmaximum for these reimbursement rates. USDA also establishes a "maximum [reimbursement] rate" intended to ensure that states distribute federal funding to all participating school food authorities relatively equally.

price is set by the school but must comply with federal regulations.[30] (Reimbursements are approximately 30 cents per lunch served).

The above reimbursement rates are approximate; exact current-year federal reimbursement rates for NSLP and SBP are listed in Table B.1 and Table B.3, respectively.

Households complete paper or online applications that collect relevant income and household size data, so that the school district can determine if children in the household are eligible for free meals, reduced-price meals, or neither.

Though these income guidelines primarily influence funding and administration of NSLP and SBP, they also affect the eligibility rules for the SFSP, CACFP, and SMP (described further in subsequent sections).

Table 2. Income Eligibility Guidelines for a Family of Four for NSLP and SBP for 48 states and DC, school year 20 1 8-20 1 9

Meal Type	Income Eligibility Threshold (% of the Federal Poverty Level)	Annual Income for a Family of Four
Free	<130%	<$32,630
Reduced-Price	130-185%	$32,630 - $46,435

Source: USDA, Food and Nutrition Service, "Child Nutrition Programs: Income Eligibility Guidelines," 83 Federal Register 20788, May 8, 2018.

Note: This school year is defined as July 1, 2018, through June 30, 2019. For other years, household sizes, Alaska, and Hawaii, see USDA-FNS website: http://www.fns.usda.gov/school-meals/income-eligibility-guidelines.

Categorical Eligibility

In addition to the eligibility thresholds listed above, the school meals programs also convey eligibility for free meals based on household participation in certain other need-tested programs or children's specified vulnerabilities (e.g., foster children). Per Section 12 of the National School

[30] The 2010 reauthorization established a policy intended to assure that paid meal revenues were covering the costs of producing a meal. See FNS paid lunch equity guidance for SY2018-2019, https://www.fns.usda.gov/school-meals/paidlunch-equity-guidance-school-year-2018-19.

Lunch Act, "a child shall be considered automatically eligible for a free lunch and breakfast ... without further application or eligibility determination, if the child is"[31]

- in a household receiving benefits through
  - SNAP (Supplemental Nutrition Assistance Program);
  - FDPIR (Food Distribution Program on Indian Reservations, a program that operates in lieu of SNAP on some Indian reservations) benefits; or
  - TANF (Temporary Assistance for Needy Families) cash assistance;
- enrolled in Head Start;
- in foster care;
- a migrant;
- a runaway; or
- homeless.[32]

For meals served to students certified in the above categories, the state/school receive a reimbursement at the free meal amount and children receive a free meal. (See Table B.1 and Table B.3 for school year 2018-2019 rates).

---

[31] See Section 9(b)(12)(A) of the Russell National School Lunch Act, codified at 42 U.S.C. 1758(b)(12)(A), for the more specific definitions of these categories.

[32] SNAP, FDPIR, and TANF have income limits, but the other qualifications, as defined, in the statute, are not limited by income. In addition to the above list, following specific demonstration authority in HHFKA as well as under FNS's standing pilot authority, some states are currently directly certifying children based on Medicaid data. According to USDA-FNS, 19 states are operating direct certification with Medicaid in SY2018-2019. Four of the states (Illinois, Kentucky, New York, Pennsylvania) use Medicaid to directly certify for free meals only. Fifteen states (California, Connecticut, Florida, Indiana, Iowa, Massachusetts, Michigan, Nebraska, Nevada, Texas, Utah, Virginia, Washington, West Virginia, Wisconsin), operating under an expanded direct certification demonstration project to test direct certification with Medicaid for reduced-price meals (up to 185% of poverty), are using this process for free and reduced-price meals. Both options are discussed in USDA-FNS, Request for Applications to Participate in Demonstration Projects to Evaluate Direct Certification with Medicaid, January 27, 2016, http://www.fns.usda.gov/sites/default/files/cn/SP23-2016a.pdf.

Some school districts collect information for these categorical eligibility rules via paper application. Others conduct a process called direct certification—a proactive process where government agencies typically cross-check their program rolls and certify a household's children for free school meals without the household having to complete a school meals application.

Prior to 2004, states had the option to conduct direct certification of SNAP (then, the Food Stamp Program), TANF, and FDPIR participants. In the 2004 child nutrition reauthorization (P.L. 108 265), states were required under federal law to conduct direct certification for SNAP participants, with nationwide implementation taking effect in school year 2008-2009. Conducting direct certification for TANF and FDPIR remains at the state's discretion.

The Healthy, Hunger-Free Kids Act of 2010 (HHFKA; P.L. 111-296) made further policy changes to expand direct certification (discussed further in the next section). One of those changes was the initiation of a demonstration project to look at expanding categorical eligibility and direct certification to some Medicaid households. The law also funded performance incentive grants for high-performing states and authorized correcting action planning for low-performing states in direct certification activities.[33]

Under SNAP direct certification rules generally, schools enter into agreements with SNAP agencies to certify children in SNAP households as eligible for free school meals without requiring a separate application from the family. Direct certification systems match student enrollment lists against SNAP agency records, eliminating the need for action by the child's parents or guardians. Direct certification allows schools to make use of SNAP's more in-depth eligibility certification process; this can reduce errors that may occur in school lunch application eligibility procedures that are otherwise used.[34] From a program access perspective,

---

[33] See CRS Report R41354, *Child Nutrition and WIC Reauthorization: P.L. 111-296*, for further discussion of these and related policies.

[34] See, for example, U.S. Government Accountability Office, *School-Meals Programs: USDA Has Enhanced Controls, but Additional Verification Could Help Ensure Legitimate*

direct certification also reduces the number of applications a household must complete.

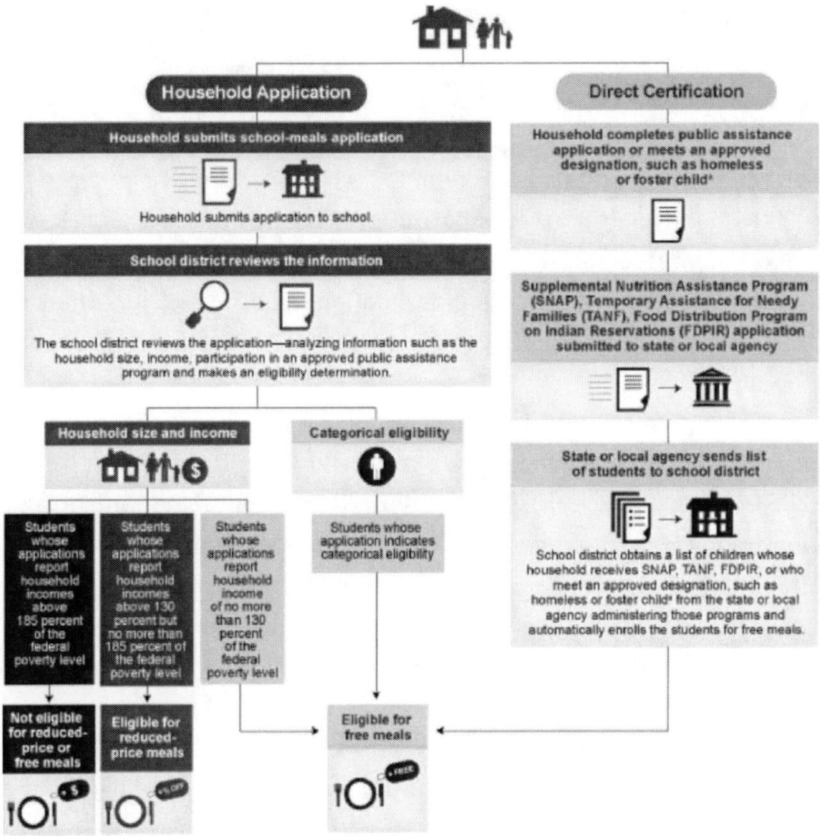

Source: GAO analysis of U.S. Department of Agriculture (USDA) information. ART Explosion (images).

Source: Figure and figure notes (below) from Government Accountability Office (GAO), GAO-14-262, p. 13.

Note: [a]Students who meet an approved designation—(1) homeless, runaway, or migrant; (2) foster child; or (3) enrolled in a federally funded Head Start Program—are categorically eligible for free school meals.

Figure 2. Overview of Certification for Free and Reduced-Price School Meals Household Application and Direct Certification Pathways.

Program Access, GAO-14-262, May 2014, pp. 16-19, http://www.gao.gov/products/GAO-14-262.

Figure 2, created by GAO and published in a May 2014 report, provides an overview of how school districts certify students for free and reduced-price meals under the income-based and category-based rules, via applications and direct certification.[35] A USDA-FNS study of school year 2014-2015 estimates that 11.1 million students receiving free meals were directly certified— 68% of all categorically eligible students receiving free meals.[36]

Community Eligibility Provision (CEP)

HHFKA also authorized the school meals Community Eligibility Provision (CEP), an option in NSLP and SBP law that allows eligible schools and school districts to offer *free meals to all enrolled students* based on the percentage of their students who are identified as automatically eligible from nonhousehold application sources (primarily direct certification through other programs).[37]

Based on the statutory parameters, USDA-FNS piloted CEP in various states over three school years and it expanded nationwide in school year 2014-2015. Eligible LEAs have until June 30 of each year to notify USDA-FNS if they will participate in CEP.[38] According to a database maintained by the Food Research and Action Center, just over 20,700 schools in more than 3,500 school districts (LEAs) participated in CEP in

---

[35] U.S. Government Accountability Office, *School-Meals Programs: USDA Has Enhanced Controls, but Additional Verification Could Help Ensure Legitimate Program Access*, GAO-14-262, May 2014, http://www.gao.gov/products/ GAO-14-262.

[36] Quinn Moore, Kevin Conway, and Brandon Kyler, et al., *Direct Certification in the National School Lunch Program: State Implementation Progress, School Year 2014-2015, Report to Congress* Mathematica Policy Research for USDA-FNS, CN-15-DC, October 2016, p. 24, https://www.fns.usda.gov/direct-certification-national-school-lunchprogram-report-congress-state-implementation-progress-0

[37] Explanation here draws in part from Madeleine Levin and Zoe Neuberger, *Improving Direct Certification Will Help More Low-Income Children Receive School Meals*, Center on Budget and Policy Priorities & Food Research and Action Center, July 25, 2014, p. 3. Aside from CEP, schools may also provide universal free meal service through the "Provision 2" and "Provision 3" options. CEP is unique in that no school meal applications are required. For information on other options, see USDA-FNS website, http://www.fns.usda.gov/school-meals/provisions-1-2-and-3.

[38] USDA Food and Nutrition Service, "National School Lunch Program and School Breakfast Program: Eliminating Applications through Community Eligibility as Required by the Healthy, Hunger-Free Kids Act of 2010," 81 *Federal Register* 50194, July 29, 2016.

SY2016-2017, an increase of approximately 2,500 schools compared to SY2015-2016.[39]

For a school (or school district, or group of schools within a district) to provide free meals to all children

- the school(s) must be eligible for CEP based on the share (40% or greater) of enrolled children that can be identified as categorically (or automatically) eligible for free meals, and
- the school must *opt-in* to CEP.

Though CEP schools serve free meals to all students, they are not reimbursed at the "free meal" rate for every meal. Instead, the law provides a funding formula: the percentage of students identified as automatically eligible (the "identified student percentage" or ISP) is multiplied by a factor of 1.6 to estimate the proportion of students who would be eligible for free or reduced-price meals had they been certified via application.[40] The result is the percentage of meals served that will be reimbursed at the free meal rate, with the remainder reimbursed at the far lower paid meal rate. For example, if a CEP school identifies that 40% of students are eligible for free meals, then 64% of the meals served will be reimbursed at the free meal rate and 36% at the paid meal rate.[41] Schools that identify 62.5% or more students as eligible for free meals receive the free meal reimbursement for all meals served.

Some of the considerations that may impact a school's decision to participate in CEP include whether the new funding formula would be beneficial for their school meal budget; an interest in reducing paperwork for families and schools; and an interest in providing more free meals,

[39] FRAC, "Community Eligibility," available at http://frac.org/community-eligibility.

[40] USDA-FNS, "National School Lunch Program and School Breakfast Program: Eliminating Applications Through Community Eligibility as Required by the Healthy, Hunger-Free Kids Act of 2010," 81 *Federal Register* 50194, July 29, 2016, p. 50201.

[41] Though, to the children of community eligibility schools, all meals are free, the USDA-FNS school meals expenditure data used throughout this chapter count these meals served in a more nuanced fashion. The percentage derived through this calculation is used to record those meals that are "free" and those meals that are "paid" (i.e., using the example from above, USDA-FNS data would reflect 64% of the meals served in the school as a "free" expenditure and meal served, and 36% as "paid").

including meals to students who have not participated in the program before.

Nutrition Standards

School Meals

The Healthy, Hunger-Free Kids Act of 2010 (HHFKA; P.L. 111-296) set in motion changes to the nutrition standards for school meals, requiring USDA to update the standards within a certain timeframe.[42] The law required that the revised standards be based on recommendations from the Institute of Medicine (IOM) (now the Health and Medicine Division) at the National Academy of Sciences. The law also provided increased federal subsidies (6 cents per lunch) for schools meeting the new requirements and funding for technical assistance related to implementation.

USDA published the final regulations in January 2012.[43] The final rule sought to align school meal patterns with the 2010 Dietary Guidelines for Americans, and, generally consistent with IOM's recommendations, increased the amount of fruits, vegetables, whole grains, and low-fat or fat-free milk in school meals. The regulations also included calorie maximums and sodium limits to phase in over time, among other requirements.

The nutrition standards largely took effect in SY2012-2013 for lunches and in SY2013-2014 for breakfasts. A few other requirements were

---

[42] The 2010 law added a deadline, but it was the 2004 reauthorization (P.L. 108-265) that required USDA to update the standards based on National Academy of Sciences recommendations. The Institute of Medicine's (IOM's) report, issued in 2010, had made a number of recommendations around such topics as imposing calorie limits, increasing fruit and vegetables, and reducing sodium intake. IOM, *School Meals: Building Blocks for Healthy Children*, Washington, DC, 2010.

[43] See 7 C.F.R. 210.10 or USDA-FNS, "Nutrition Standards in the National School Lunch and School Breakfast Programs," 77 *Federal Register* 17, January 26, 2012, available at https://www.federalregister.gov/documents/2012/01/ 26/2012-1010/nutrition-standards-in-the-national-school-lunch-and-school-breakfast-programs. For related resources, see USDA-FNS website at http://www.fns.usda.gov/school-meals/nutrition-standards-school-meals.

scheduled to phase in over multiple school years.[44] Some schools experienced difficulty implementing the new guidelines, and Congress and USDA have made changes to the 2012 final rule's whole grain, sodium, and milk requirements.[45] For SY2019-2020 and onwards, schools are operating under a final rule published December 12, 2018.[46]

Competitive Foods

The HHFKA also gave USDA the authority to regulate other foods in the school nutrition environment. Sometimes called "competitive foods," these include foods and drinks sold in a la carte lines, vending machines, snack bars and concession stands, and fundraisers.

Relying on recommendations made by a 2007 IOM report, USDA-FNS promulgated a proposed rule and then an interim final rule in June 2013, which went into effect for SY2014-2015.[47] The interim final rule created nutrition guidelines for all non-meal foods and beverages that are sold *during the school day* (defined as midnight until 30 minutes after dismissal). The final rule, published on July 29, 2016, maintained the interim final rules with minor modifications.[48] Under the final standards, these foods must meet whole-grain requirements; have certain primary ingredients; and meet calorie, sodium, and fat limits, among other

---

[44] For the original implementation schedule based on the January 2012 final rule, see USDA-FNS Implementation Timeline, http://www.fns.usda.gov/sites/default/files/implementation_timeline.pdf.

[45] For more information, see CRS Report R45486, *Child Nutrition Programs: Current Issues*.

[46] USDA-FNS, "Child Nutrition Programs: Flexibilities for Milk, Whole Grains, and Sodium Requirements: Final Rule," 83 *Federal Register* 63775, December 12, 2018, available at https://www.federalregister.gov/documents/2018/12/12/2018-26762/child-nutrition-programs-flexibilities-for-milk-whole-grains-and-sodium-requirements.

[47] IOM, *Nutrition Standards for Foods in Schools: Leading the Way toward Healthier Youth*, 2007, https://www.nap.edu/catalog/11899/nutrition-standards-for-foods-in-schools-leading-the-way-toward; USDA-FNS, "Interim Rule: NSLP and SBP Nutrition Standards for All Foods Sold in Schools as Required by the Healthy, Hunger-Free Kids Act of 2010," 78 *Federal Register* 79567, December 31, 2013, available at https://www.federalregister.gov/documents/2013/12/31/2013-31350/national-school-lunch-program-and-school-breakfast-program-nutrition-standards-for-all-foods-sold-in.

[48] USDA-FNS, "National School Lunch Program and School Breakfast Program: Nutrition Standards for All Foods Sold in School as Required by the Healthy, Hunger-Free Kids Act of 2010; Final Rule," 81 *Federal Register* 50131, July 29, 2016. The final rule and related resources are available at the USDA-FNS website, https://www.fns.usda.gov/ school-meals/tools-schools-focusing-smart-snacks.

requirements. Schools are limited to a list of no- and low-calorie beverages they may sell (with larger portion sizes and caffeine allowed in high schools).

There are no limits on fundraisers selling foods that meet the interim final rule's guidelines. Fundraisers outside of the school day are not subject to the guidelines. HHFKA and the interim final rule provide states with discretion to exempt infrequent fundraisers selling foods or beverages that do not meet the nutrition standards.

The rule does not limit foods brought from home, only foods sold at school during the school day. The federal standards are minimum standards; states and school districts are permitted to issue more stringent policies.

National School Lunch Program (NSLP)

In FY2017, NSLP subsidized 4.9 billion lunches to children in close to 96,000 schools and 3,200 residential child care institutions (RCCIs). Average daily participation was 30.0 million students (58% of children enrolled in participating schools and RCCIs). Of the participating students, 66.7% (20.0 million) received free lunches and 6.5% (2.0 million) received reduced-price lunches. The remainder were served full-price meals, though schools still receive a reimbursement for these meals. Figure 3 shows FY2017 participation data.

FY2017 federal school lunch costs totaled approximately $13.6 billion (see Table 3 for the various components of this total). The vast majority of this funding is for per-meal reimbursements for free and reduced-price lunches.

The HHFKA also provided an additional 6-cent per-lunch reimbursement to schools that provide meals that meet the updated nutritional guidelines requirements.[49] This bonus is not provided for

[49] In January 2014, USDA-FNS issued a final rule implementing the 6-cent reimbursement: USDA-FNS, "Certification of Compliance With Meal Requirements for the National School Lunch Program Under the Healthy, Hunger-Free Kids Act of 2010," 79 *Federal*

breakfast, but funds may be used to support schools' breakfast programs. NSLP lunch reimbursement rates are listed in Table B.1.

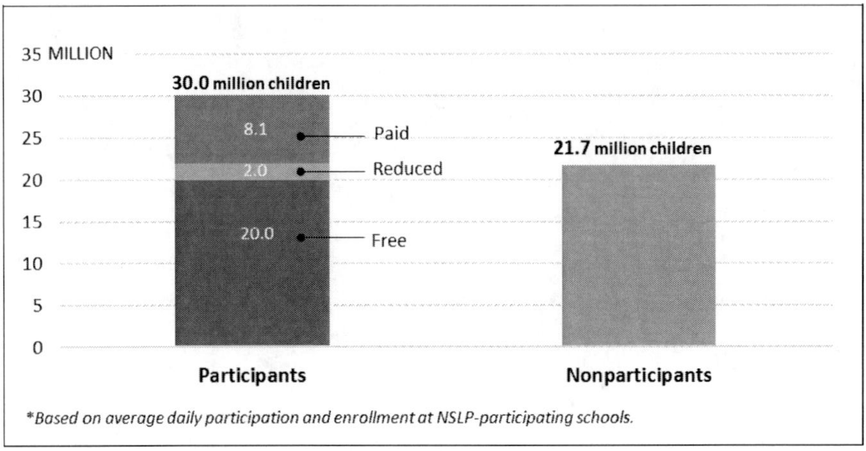

Source: Figure created by CRS based on FY2017 data from the USDA-FNS Key data May 2018 report.

Notes: Numbers may not add due to rounding. To reflect participation for the actual school year (September through May), these estimates are based on nine-month averages of October through May plus September, rather than averages of the 12 months of the fiscal year (October through September). Participation data are estimated by USDA-FNS based on average daily meals served. Children in schools participating in the Community Eligibility Provision (CEP) are counted in the free and paid meal categories.

Figure 3. National School Lunch Program, FY2017 Participation among children at NSLP-participating schools.

In addition to federal *cash* subsidies, schools participating in NSLP receive USDA-acquired *commodity foods*. Schools are entitled to a specific, inflation-indexed value of USDA commodity foods for each lunch they serve. Also, schools may receive donations of bonus commodities acquired by USDA in support of the farm economy.[50] In FY2017, the value

---

Register 326, January 3, 2014. Note: 6-cent increase authorized is also annually indexed for inflation.

[50] USDA commodity foods are foods purchased by the USDA for distribution to USDA nutrition programs. These programs distribute "entitlement commodities" (an amount of USDA foods to which grantees are entitled by law) as well as "bonus commodities" (USDA food

of federal commodity food aid to schools totaled nearly $1.4 billion. The per-meal rate for commodity food assistance is included in Table B.4.

While the vast majority of NSLP funding is for lunches served during the school day, NSLP may also be used to support snack service during the school year and to serve meals during the summer. These features are discussed in subsequent sections, "Summer Meals" and "After-School Meals and Snacks: CACFP, NSLP Options." Reimbursement rates for snacks are listed in Table B.2.

School Breakfast Program (SBP)

The School Breakfast Program (SBP) provides per-meal cash subsidies for breakfasts served in schools. Participating schools receive subsidies based on their status as a severe need or nonsevere need institution. Schools can qualify as a severe need school if 40% or more of their lunches are served free or at reduced prices. See Table B.3 for SBP reimbursement rates.

Figure 4 displays SBP participation data for FY2017. In that year, SBP subsidized over 2.4 billion breakfasts in over 88,000 schools and nearly 3,200 RCCIs. Average daily participation was 14.7 million children (30.1% of the students enrolled in participating schools and RCCIs). The majority of meals served through SBP are free or reduced-price. Of the participating students, 79.1% (11.6 million) received free meals and 5.7% (835,000) purchased reduced-price meals. Federal school breakfast costs for the fiscal year totaled approximately $4.3 billion (see Table 3 for the various components of this total).

Significantly fewer schools and students participate in SBP than in NSLP. Participation in SBP tends to be lower for several reasons, including the traditionally required early arrival by students in order to receive a meal and eat before school starts. Some schools offer (and anti-hunger groups have encouraged) models of breakfast service that can result

---

purchases based on requests from the agricultural producer community). For more information see CRS Report R42353, *Domestic Food Assistance: Summary of Programs*.

in greater SBP participation, such as Breakfast in the Classroom, where meals are delivered in the classroom; "grab and go" carts, where students receive a bagged breakfast that they bring to class, or serving breakfast later in the day in middle and high schools.[51]

Unlike NSLP, commodity food assistance is not a formal part of SBP funding; however, commodities provided through NSLP may be used for school breakfasts as well.

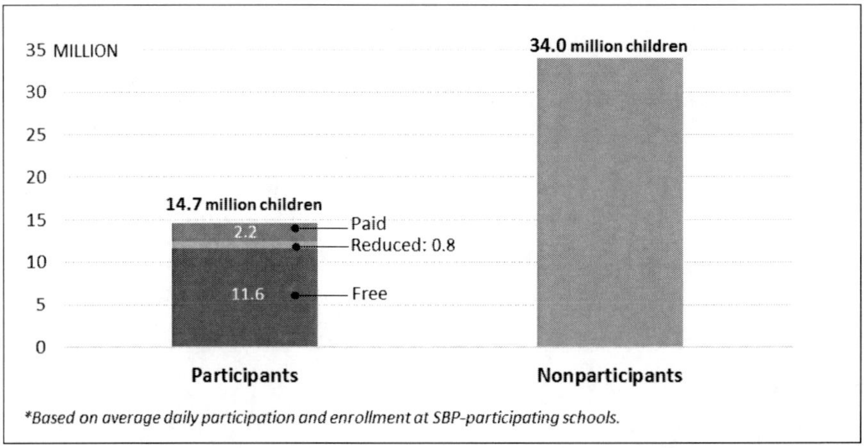

Source: Figure created by CRS based on FY2017 data from the USDA-FNS Key data May 2018 report.

Notes: Numbers may not add due to rounding. To reflect participation for the actual school year (September through May), these estimates are based on nine-month averages of October through May plus September, rather than averages of the 12 months of the fiscal year (October through September). Participation data are estimated by USDA-FNS based on average daily meals served. Children in schools participating in the Community Eligibility Provision (CEP) are counted in the free and paid meal categories.

Figure 4. School Breakfast Program, FY2017 Participation among children at SBP-participating schools.

---

[51] See Food Research and Action Center (FRAC), "School Breakfast Expansion Strategies," http://www.frac.org/ programs/school-breakfast-program/school-breakfast-expansion-strategies (accessed July 9, 2018).

OTHER CHILD NUTRITION PROGRAMS

In addition to the school meals programs discussed above, other federal child nutrition programs provide federal subsidies and commodity food assistance for schools and other institutions that offer meals and snacks to children in early childhood, summer, and after-school settings. This assistance is provided to (1) schools and other governmental institutions, (2) private for-profit and nonprofit child care centers, (3) family/group day care homes, and (4) nongovernmental institutions/organizations that offer outside-of-school programs for children. (Although this chapter focuses on the programs that serve children, one child nutrition program (CACFP) also serves day care centers for chronically impaired adults and elderly persons under the same general per meal/snack subsidy terms.) The programs in the sections to follow serve comparatively fewer children and spend comparatively fewer federal funds than the school meal programs.

Child and Adult Care Food Program (CACFP)

CACFP subsidizes meals and snacks served in early childhood, day care, and after-school settings. CACFP provides subsidies for meals and snacks served at participating nonresidential child care centers, family day care homes, and (to a lesser extent) adult day care centers.[52] The program also provides assistance for meals served at after-school programs. CACFP reimbursements are available for meals and snacks served to children age 12 or under, migrant children age 15 or under, children with disabilities of any age, and, in the case of adult care centers, chronically impaired and elderly adults.

---

[52] CACFP also supports meals in homeless/emergency shelters. See http://www.fns.usda.gov/cacfp/emergency-shelters for further information.

Children in early childhood settings are the overwhelming majority of those served by the program. CACFP provides federal reimbursements for breakfasts, lunches, suppers, and snacks served in participating centers (facilities or institutions) or day care homes (private homes). The eligibility and funding rules for CACFP meals and snacks depend first on whether the participating institution is a center or a day care home (the next two sections discuss the rules specific to centers and day care homes). According to FY2017 CACFP data, child care centers have an average daily attendance of about 56 children per center, day care homes have an average daily attendance of approximately 7 children per home, and adult day care centers typically care for an average of 48 chronically ill or elderly adults per center.[53]

Providers must demonstrate that they comply with government-established standards for other child care programs. Like in school meals, federal assistance is made up overwhelmingly of *cash* reimbursements calculated based on the number of meals/snacks served and federal per-meal/snack reimbursements rates, but a far smaller share of federal aid (4.3% in FY2017) is in the form of federal USDA commodity *foods* (or cash in lieu of foods). Federal CACFP reimbursements flow to individual providers either directly from the administering state agency (this is the case with many child/adult care centers able to handle their own CACFP administrative functions) or through "sponsors" who oversee and provide administrative support for a number of local providers (this is the case with some child/adult care centers and with all day care homes).[54]

In FY2017, total CACFP spending was over $3.5 billion, including cash reimbursement, commodity food assistance, and costs for sponsor audits. (See Table 3 for a further breakdown of CACFP costs.)

---

[53] USDA-FNS' administrative data on the CACFP are the source of these attendance numbers.

[54] In many cases, sponsor organizations that provide administrative support to multiple providers also are paid federal reimbursements for their costs. Day care homes must have a sponsoring organization, while child care centers may have a sponsor but are not required to do so.

This total also includes the after-school meals and snacks provided through CACFP's "at-risk after-school" pathway; this aspect of the program is discussed later in "After-School Meals and Snacks: CACFP, NSLP Options."

Table 3. FY2016 and FY2017 Federal Expenditures on Child Nutrition Programs, In millions of dollars

Program or Program Component	FY2016	FY2017	Change from FY2016 to FY2017	
National School Lunch Program	$13,569	$13,643	+$74	+1%
free meal reimbursements	$9,593	$9,620	+$27	0%
reduced-price meal reimbursements	$808	$783	-$25	-3%
paid meal reimbursements	$1,478	$1,480	+$2	0%
additional funding to schools with more than 60% free or reduced price participation	$76	$74	-$2	-3%
performance-based meal reimbursements	$302	$293	-$9	-3%
commodity food assistance[a]	$1,311	$1,393	+$82	+6%
School Breakfast Program	$4,213	$4,252	+$39	+1%
free meal reimbursements	$3,868	$3,912	+$44	+1%
reduced-price meal reimbursements	$239	$235	-$4	-2%
paid meal reimbursements	$106	$106	$0	0%
Child and Adult Care Food Program	$3,520	$3,537	+$17	0%
meal reimbursements at child care centers	$2,307	$2,363	+$56	+2%
meal reimbursements at child care homes	$764	$721	-$42	-6%
meal reimbursements at adult day care centers	$149	$156	+$7	+5%
commodity food assistance[a]	$155	$153	-$2	-1%
administrative costs for child care sponsors	$146	$145	-$1	-1%
Summer Food Service Program	$478	$485	+$7	+1%
meal reimbursements	$419	$424	+$5	+1%
commodity food assistance[a]	$2	$2	$0	0%
sponsor and inspection costs	$58	$60	+$2	+3%
Special Milk Program	$9	$8	-$1	-11%
Fresh Fruit and Vegetable Program[b]	$167	$184	+$17	+10%
State Administrative Expenses	$260	$279	+$19	+7%
Mandatory Other Program Costs[c]	$59	$83	+$24	+41%

Table 3. (Continued)

Program or Program Component	FY2016	FY2017	Change from FY2016 to FY2017	
Discretionary Activities[d]	$69	$63	-$6	-9%
TOTAL OF FUNDS DISPLAYED[e]	$22,344	$22,534	+$192	+1%

Source: Program expenditures data (outlays) from USDA-FNS Key data Reports (dated March 2017 and March 2018), except where noted below.

Notes: Expenditures displayed here will vary from displays in CRS appropriations reports and in some cases the USDA-FNS annual budget justification. Since the majority of program funding is for open-ended entitlements, expenditure data capture spending better than the total of appropriations. This table includes some functions that are funded through permanent appropriations or transfers (i.e., funding not provided in appropriations laws). Due to rounding to the nearest million, percentage increases or decreases may be exaggerated or understated.

a. Amounts included in this table for commodity food assistance include only entitlement commodities for each program, not bonus commodities.

b. Obligations data displayed on p. 32-14 of FY2019 USDA-FNS Congressional Budget Justification.

c. Obligations data displayed on p. 32-12 of FY2019 USDA-FNS Congressional Budget Justification. These costs are made up of Food Safety Education, Coordinated Review, Computer Support, Training and Technical Assistance, studies, payment accuracy, and Farm to School Team.

d. Obligations data displayed on p. 32-12 of FY2019 USDA-FNS Congressional Budget Justification. These costs include Team Nutrition, the Summer EBT demonstration, and School Meal Equipment Grants.

e. This table summarizes the vast majority of child nutrition programs' federal spending but does not capture all federal costs.

CACFP Nutrition Standards

As with school foods, the HHFKA required USDA to update CACFP's meal patterns. USDA's final rule revised the meal patterns for both meals served in child care centers and day care homes, as well as preschool meals served through the NSLP and SBP, effective October 1, 2017.[55] For infants (under 12 months of age), the new meal patterns eliminated juice, supported breastfeeding, and set guidelines for the introduction of solid foods, among other changes. For children ages one and older, the new meal patterns increased whole grains, fruits and vegetables, and low-fat and fat-

[55] USDA-FNS, "Child and Adult Care Food Program: Meal Pattern Revisions Related to the Healthy, Hunger-Free Kids Act of 2010; Final Rule," 81 *Federal Register* 24348 et seq., April 25, 2016, https://www.federalregister.gov/ documents/2016/04/25/2016-09412/child-and-adult-care-food-program-meal-pattern-revisions-related-to-the-healthyhunger-free-kids-act.

free milk; limited sugar in cereals and yogurts; and prohibited frying, among other requirements.

CACFP at Centers Participation

Child care centers in CACFP can be (1) public or private nonprofit centers, (2) Head Start centers, (3) for-profit proprietary centers (if they meet certain requirements as to the proportion of low-income children they enroll), and (4) shelters for homeless families. Adult day care centers include public or private nonprofit centers and for-profit proprietary centers (if they meet minimum requirements related to serving low-income disabled and elderly adults).[56] In FY2017, over 65,000 child care centers with an average daily attendance of over 3.6 million children participated in CACFP. Over 2,700 adult care centers served nearly 132,000 adults through CACFP.

Eligibility and Administration

Participating centers may receive daily reimbursements for up to either two meals and one snack or one meal and two snacks for each participant, so long as the meals and snacks meet federal nutrition standards.

The eligibility rules for CACFP centers largely track those of NSLP: children in households at or below 130% of the current poverty line qualify for free meals/snacks while those between 130% and 185% of poverty qualify for reduced-price meals/snacks (see Table 2). In addition, participation in the same categorical eligibility programs as NSLP as well as foster child status convey eligibility for free meals in CACFP.[57] Like school meals, eligibility is determined through paper applications or direct certification processes.

Like school meals, all meals and snacks served in the centers are federally subsidized to some degree, even those that are paid. Different

---

[56] Participating adult care programs "should be structured, comprehensive and provide health and social support services to enrolled participants. Centers that simply provide social or rehabilitative services to adults do not qualify to participate in CACFP." http://www.fns.usda.gov/cacfp/facts-about-adult-component-cacfp.

[57] See also summary of CACFP eligibility rules at USDA-FNS website, http://www.fns.usda.gov/cacfp/why-cacfpimportant.

reimbursement amounts are provided for breakfasts, lunches/suppers, and snacks, and reimbursement rates are set in law and indexed for inflation annually. The largest subsidies are paid for meals and snacks served to participants with family income below 130% of the federal poverty income guidelines (the income limit for free school meals), and the smallest to those who have not met a means test. See Table B.5 for current CACFP center reimbursement rates.

Unlike school meals, CACFP institutions are less likely to collect per-meal payments. Although federal assistance for day care centers differentiates by household income, centers have discretion on their pricing of meals. Centers may adjust their regular fees (tuition) to account for federal payments, but CACFP itself does not regulate these fees. In addition, centers can charge families separately for meals/snacks, so long as there are no charges for children meeting free-meal/snack income tests and limited charges for those meeting reduced-price income tests.

Independent centers are those without sponsors handling administrative responsibilities. These centers must pay for administrative costs associated with CACFP out of nonfederal funds or a portion of their meal subsidy payments. For centers with sponsors, the sponsors may retain a proportion of the meal reimbursement payments they receive on behalf of their centers to cover such costs.

CACFP for Day Care Homes

Participation

CACFP-supported day care *homes* serve a smaller number of children than CACFP-supported *centers*, both in terms of the total number of children served and the average number of children per facility. Roughly 17% of children in CACFP (approximately 757,000 in FY2017 average daily attendance) are served through day care homes. In FY2017, approximately 103,000 homes (with just over 700 sponsors) received CACFP support.

Eligibility and Reimbursement

As with centers, payments to day care homes are provided for up to either two meals and one snack or one meal and two snacks a day for each child. Unlike centers, day care homes must participate under the auspices of a public or, more often, private nonprofit sponsor that typically has 100 or more homes under its supervision. CACFP day care home sponsors receive monthly administrative payments based on the number of homes for which they are responsible.[58]

Federal reimbursements for family day care homes differ by the home's status as "Tier I" or "Tier II." Unlike centers, day care homes receive cash reimbursements (but not commodity foods) that generally are not based on the child participants' household income. Instead, there are two distinct, annually indexed reimbursement rates that are based on area or operator eligibility criteria

- Tier I homes are located in low-income areas (defined as areas in which at least 50% of school-age and enrolled children qualify for free or reduced-price meals) or operated by low-income providers whose household income meets the free or reduced-price income standards.[59] They receive higher subsidies for each meal/snack they serve.
- Tier II (lower) rates are by default those for homes that do not qualify for Tier I rates; however, Tier II providers may seek the higher Tier I subsidy rates for individual low-income children for whom financial information is collected and verified. (See Table B.6 for current Tier I and Tier II reimbursement rates).

---

[58] As an example of the role that sponsors and homes play in CACFP, in Allentown, Pennsylvania, the Lehigh Valley Children's Centers (LVCC) serves as a sponsor for child care homes in the area. They offer a variety of administrative services to family child care homes that are registered with the state. In their brochure, they state that it is LVCC's responsibility to "monitor meals and reimburse [homes] for meals served," and it is homes' responsibility "to plan nutritional menus that meet meal requirements, maintain and submit daily attendance records and monthly meal counts." See http://www.lvcconline.org/images/pdf/CACFP-Brochure.pdf.

[59] 7 C.F.R. §226.2.

Additionally, HHFKA introduced a number of additional ways (as compared to prior law) by which family day care homes can qualify as low-income and get Tier I rates for the entire home or for individual children.[60]

As with centers, there is no requirement that meals/snacks specifically identified as free or reduced-price be offered; however, unlike centers, federal rules prohibit any separate meal charges.

Summer Meals

Current law SFSP and the NSLP/SBP Seamless Summer Option provide meals in congregate settings nationwide; the related Summer Electronic Benefits Transfer (SEBTC or Summer EBT) demonstration project is an alternative to congregate settings.

Summer Food Service Program (SFSP)

SFSP supports meals for children during the summer months. The program provides assistance to local public institutions and private nonprofit service institutions running summer youth/recreation programs, summer feeding projects, and camps. Assistance is primarily in the form of cash reimbursements for each meal or snack served; however, federally donated commodity foods are also offered. Participating service

---

[60] Previously, child care homes could only use data from the elementary school level to establish the area as low-income. The new law allows these homes to use data from the middle and high school level as well to establish need and qualify as a "Tier I" home. Also, P.L. 111-296 included policies to streamline application processes and eliminate some paperwork. As part of this process, the annual application process has been eliminated and sponsors and child care centers will only have to submit paperwork the first time they apply, with amendments submitted as necessary. Finally, P.L. 111-296 increased CACFP sponsoring organizations' and providers' flexibility over administrative funds, including the option to carry over up to 10% of administrative funds from one fiscal year to the next. USDA-FNS has begun to implement these changes. See, for example, USDA Food and Nutrition Service, "Child and Adult Care Food Program: Amendments Related to the Healthy, Hunger-Free Kids Act of 2010," 77 *Federal Register* 21018-21038, April 9, 2012; USDA-FNS Memorandum, *Child Nutrition Reauthorization 2010: Area Eligibility for Family Day Care Homes*, Memo Code: CACFP 05-2011-Revised, January 10, 2011, https://www.fns.usda.gov/cacfp-05-2011-revisedchild-nutrition-reauthorization-2010-area-eligibility-family-day-care-homes.

institutions are often entities that provide ongoing year-round service to the community including schools, local governments, camps, colleges and universities in the National Youth Sports program, and private nonprofit organizations like churches.

Similar to the CACFP model, sponsors are institutions that manage the food preparation, financial, and administrative responsibilities of SFSP. Sites are the places where food is served and eaten. At times, a sponsor may also be a site. State agencies authorize sponsors, monitor and inspect sponsors and sites, and implement USDA policy. Unlike CACFP, sponsors are required for an institution's participation in SFSP as a site.

Participation

In FY2017, nearly 5,500 sponsors with 50,000 food service sites participated in the SFSP and served an average of approximately 2.7 million children daily (according to July data).[61]

Participation of sites and children in SFSP has increased in recent years. Program costs for FY2017 totaled over $485 million, including cash assistance, commodity foods, administrative cost assistance, and health inspection costs.

Eligibility and Administration

There are several options for eligibility and meal/snack service for SFSP sponsors (and their sites)

- Open sites provide summer food to all children in the community. These sites are certified based on *area* eligibility measures, where 50% or more of area children have family income that would make them eligible for free or reduced-price school meals (see Table 2).
- Closed or Enrolled sites provide summer meals/snacks free to all children enrolled at the site. The eligibility test for these sites is

[61] According to a May 2018 GAO report, estimates of participation in SFSP may not be reliable because they have been calculated inconsistently across states and years. See U.S. Government Accountability Office, *Actions Needed to Improve Participation Estimates and Address Program Challenges,* GAO-18-369, May 2018, https://www.gao.gov/products/GAO-18-369.

that 50% or more of the *children enrolled* in the sponsor's program must be eligible for free or reduced-price school meals based on household income. Closed/enrolled sites may also become eligible based on area eligibility measures noted above.

- Summer camps (that are not enrolled sites) receive subsidies only for those children with household eligibility for free or reduced-price school meals.
- Other programs specified in law, such as the National Youth Sports Program and centers for homeless or migrant children.

Summer sponsors get operating cost (food, storage, labor) subsidies for all meals/snacks they serve—up to one meal and one snack, or two meals per child per day.[62] In addition, sponsors receive payments for administrative costs, and states are provided with subsidies for administrative costs and health and meal-quality inspections. See Table B.7 for current SFSP reimbursement rates. Actual payments vary slightly (e.g., by about 5 cents for lunches) depending on the location of the site (e.g., rural vs. urban) and whether meals are prepared on-site or by a vendor.

School Meals' Seamless Summer Option[63]

Although SFSP is the child nutrition program most associated with providing meals during summer months, it is not the only program option for providing these meals and snacks. The Seamless Summer Option, run through NSLP or SBP programs, is also a means through which food can be provided to students during summer months. Much like SFSP, Seamless Summer operates in summer *sites* (summer camps, sports programs, churches, private nonprofit organizations, etc.) and for a similar duration of time. Unlike SFSP, *schools are the only eligible sponsors*, although

---

[62] With state agency approval, camps and migrant sites (sites that predominantly serve children of migrant workers) may be reimbursed for serving three meals or two meals and one snack per child daily.

[63] For further discussion, see the USDA-FNS website: http://www.fns.usda.gov/school-meals/opportunity-schools.

schools may operate the program at other sites. Reimbursement rates for Seamless Summer meals are the same as current NSLP/SBP rates.

Summer EBT for Children Demonstration

Beginning in summer 2011 and (as of the date of this chapter) each summer since, USDA-FNS has operated Summer Electronic Benefit Transfer for Children (SEBTC or "Summer EBT") demonstration projects in a limited number of states and Indian Tribal Organizations (ITOs). These Summer EBT projects provide electronic food benefits over summer months to households with children eligible for free or reduced-price school meals. Depending on the site and year, either $30 or $60 per month is provided, through a WIC or SNAP EBT card model. In the demonstration projects, these benefits were provided as a supplement to the Summer Food Service Program (SFSP) meals available in congregate settings.

Summer EBT and other alternatives to congregate meals through SFSP were first authorized and funded by the FY2010 appropriations law (P.L. 111-80).[64] Although a number of alternatives were tested and evaluated, findings from Summer EBT were among the most promising, and Congress provided subsequent funding.[65] Summer EBT evaluations showed significant impacts on reducing child food insecurity and improving nutritional intake.[66] Summer EBT was funded by P.L. 111-80 in the summers from 2011 to 2014. Projects have continued to operate and were annually funded by FY2015-FY2018 appropriations; most recently, the FY2018 appropriations law (P.L. 115-141) provided $28 million. According to USDA-FNS, in summer 2016 Summer EBT served over 209,000 children in nine states and two tribal nations—an increase from

---

[64] For more information, see CRS Report R45486, *Child Nutrition Programs: Current Issues*.

[65] This CRS report discusses Summer EBT, not the other tested programs ("Enhanced Summer Food Service Program (eSFSP)). For information on eSFSP, see USDA-FNS' "Enhanced Summer Food Service Program" web page, https://www.fns.usda.gov/ops/enhanced-summer-food-service-program-esfsp.

[66] Collins et al., *Summer Electronic Benefits Transfer for Children (SEBTC) Demonstration: Evaluation Findings for the Full Implementation Year.* Prepared by Abt Associates, Mathematica Policy Research, and Maximus (Alexandria, VA: USDA, Food and Nutrition Service, 2013), p. 105. This improvement is based on the entire evaluation population. Improvements in VLFS-C did vary significantly between Summer EBT sites.

the 11,400 children served when the demonstration began in summer 2011.[67]

Special Milk Program (SMP)

Schools (and institutions like summer camps and child care facilities) that are not already participating in the other child nutrition programs can participate in the Special Milk Program. Schools may also administer SMP for their part-day sessions for kindergartners or pre-kindergartners.

Under SMP, participating institutions provide milk to children for free and/or at a subsidized paid price, depending on how the enrolled institution opts to administer the program (see Table B.8 for current Special Milk reimbursement rates for each of these options)

- An institution that *only sells milk* will receive the same per-half pint federal reimbursement for each milk sold (approximately 20 cents).
- An institution that *sells milk and provides free milk* to eligible children (income eligibility is the same as free school meals, see Table 2), receives a reimbursement for the milk sold (approximately 20 cents) and a higher reimbursement for the free milks.
- An institution that *does not sell milk* provides milk free to all children and receives the same reimbursement for all milk (approximately 20 cents). This option is sometimes called nonpricing.

In FY2017, over 41 million half-pints were subsidized, 9.5% of which were served free. Federal expenditures for this program were approximately $8.3 million in FY2017.

---

[67] *FY2019 USDA Budget Explanatory Notes for Committee on Appropriations* for USDA-FNS, p. 32-40, https://www.obpa.usda.gov/32fns2019notes.pdf.

Fresh Fruit and Vegetable Program (FFVP)

States receive formula grants through the Fresh Fruit and Vegetable Program, under which state-selected schools receive funds to purchase and distribute *fresh* fruit and vegetable snacks to all children in attendance (regardless of family income). Money is distributed by a formula under which about half the funding is distributed equally to each state and the remainder is allocated by state population. States select participating schools (with an emphasis on those with a higher proportion of low-income children) and set annual per-student grant amounts (between $50 and $75).

Funding is set by law at $150 million for school year 2011-2012 and inflation-indexed for every year after. In FY2017, states used approximately $184 million in FFVP funds.[68] FFVP is funded by a mandatory transfer of funds from USDA's Section 32 program—a permanent appropriation of 30% of the previous year's customs receipts.[69] This transfer is required by FFVP's authorizing laws (Section 19 of the Richard B. Russell National School Lunch Act and Section 4304 of P.L. 110-246). Up until FY2018's law, annual appropriations laws delayed a portion of the funds to the next fiscal year.

After a pilot period, the Child Nutrition and WIC Reauthorization Act of 2004 (P.L. 108-265) permanently authorized and funded FFVP for a limited number of states and Indian reservations.[70] In recent years, FFVP has been amended by omnibus farm bill laws rather than through child nutrition reauthorizations. The 2008 farm bill (P.L. 110-246) expanded FFVP's mandatory funding, specifically providing funds through Section 32, and enabled all states to participate in the program. The 2014 farm bill (P.L. 113-79) essentially made no changes to this program but did include, and fund at $5 million in FY2014, a pilot project that requires USDA to

---

[68] *FY2019 USDA Budget Explanatory Notes for Committee on Appropriations* for USDA-FNS, p. 32-14, https://www.obpa.usda.gov/32fns2019notes.pdf.

[69] For more information, see CRS Report RL34081, *Farm and Food Support Under USDA's Section 32 Program.*

[70] Permanent funding is made possible through the Section 32 account. See CRS Report RL34081, *Farm and Food Support Under USDA's Section 32 Program*, coordinated by Jim Monke.

test offering frozen, dried, and canned fruits and vegetables and publish an evaluation of the pilot. Four states (Alaska, Delaware, Kansas, and Maine) participated in the pilot in SY2014-2015 and the evaluation was published in 2017.[71] Other proposals to expand fruits and vegetables offered in FFVP have been introduced in both the 114th and 115th Congress.[72]

OTHER TOPICS

After-School Meals and Snacks: CACFP, NSLP Options

Two of the child nutrition programs discussed in previous sections, the National School Lunch Program (NSLP) and Child and Adult Care Food Program (CACFP), provide federal support for snacks and meals served during after-school programs.[73]

NSLP provides reimbursements for after-school snacks; however, this option is open only to schools that already participate in NSLP. These schools may operate after-school snack-only programs during the school year, and can do so in two ways: (1) if low-income area eligibility criteria are met, provide free snacks in lower-income areas; or (2) if area eligibility criteria are not met, offer free, reduced-price, or fully paid-for snacks, based on household income eligibility (like lunches in NSLP). The vast majority of snacks provided through this program are through the first option. Through this program, approximately 206 million snacks were served in FY2017 (a daily average of nearly 1.3 million). This compares with nearly 4.9 billion *lunches* served (a daily average of 27.8 million).

---

[71] Briefel et al., Evaluation of the Pilot Project for Canned, Frozen, or Dried Fruits and Vegetables in the Fresh Fruit and Vegetable Program (FFVP-CFD), Prepared by Mathematica Policy Research. Alexandria, VA: USDA, Food and Nutrition Service, January 2017, available at https://fns-prod.azureedge.net/sites/default/files/ops/FFVP-CFD.pdf.

[72] See CRS Report R44373, *Tracking the Next Child Nutrition Reauthorization: An Overview*. In the 115th Congress, see H.R. 3402, S. 2064, and House-passed H.R. 2 §4204.

[73] For further discussion of the NSLP and CACFP after-school snack program, see Joanne Guthrie, *Feeding Children After School: The Expanding Role of USDA Child Nutrition Programs*, USDA Economic Research Service, Amber Waves, March 1, 2012, https://www.ers.usda.gov/amber-waves/2012/march/feeding-children-after-school/.

CACFP provides assistance for after-school food in two ways. First, centers and homes that participate in CACFP and provide after-school care may participate in traditional CACFP (the eligibility and administration described earlier). Second, centers in areas where at least half the children in the community are eligible for free or reduced-price school meals can opt to participate in the CACFP At-Risk Afterschool program, which provides free snacks and suppers. Expansion of the At-Risk After-School meals program was a major policy change included in HHFKA. Prior to the law, 13 states were permitted to offer CACFP At-Risk After-School meals (instead of just a snack); the law allowed all CACFP state agencies to offer such meals.[74] In FY2017, the At-Risk Afterschool program served a total of approximately 242.6 million free meals and snacks to a daily average of more than 1.7 million children.[75]

Related Programs, Initiatives, and Support Activities

Federal child nutrition laws authorize and program funding supports a range of additional programs, initiatives, and activities.[76]

Through State Administrative Expenses funding, states are entitled to federal grants to help cover administrative and oversight/monitoring costs associated with child nutrition programs. The national amount each year is equal to about 2% of child nutrition reimbursements. The majority of this money is allocated to states based on their share of spending on the covered programs; about 15% is allocated under a discretionary formula granting each state additional amounts for CACFP, commodity distribution, and Administrative Review efforts. In addition, states receive payments for their role in overseeing summer programs (about 2.5% of their summer program aid). States are free to apportion their federal

[74] S.Rept. 111-178, p. 7.

[75] Data provided by USDA-FNS on July 18, 2018.

[76] This section does not list all related federal funding and support activities; those activities that are discussed are broadly summarized. For further details on these and other functions funded by the "child nutrition programs" account, see the *2019 USDA Budget Explanatory Notes for Committee on Appropriations* for USDA-FNS, pp. 32-10 through 32-26, https://www.obpa.usda.gov/32fns2019notes.pdf.

administrative expense payments among child nutrition initiatives (including commodity distribution activities) as they see fit, and appropriated funding is available to states for two years. State Administrative Expense spending in FY2017 totaled approximately $279 million.[77]

Team Nutrition is a USDA-FNS program that includes a variety of school meals initiatives around nutrition education and the nutritional content of the foods children eat in schools. This includes Team Nutrition Training Grants, which provide funding to state agencies for training and technical assistance, such as help implementing USDA's nutrition requirements and the Dietary Guidelines for Americans. From 2004 to 2018, Team Nutrition also included the HealthierUS Schools Challenge (HUSSC), which originated in the 2004 reauthorization of the Child Nutrition Act. HUSSC was a voluntary certification initiative designed to recognize schools that have created a healthy school environment through the promotion of nutrition and physical activity.[78]

Farm-to-school programs broadly refer to "efforts that bring regionally and locally produced foods into school cafeterias," with a focus on enhancing child nutrition.[79] The goals of these efforts include increasing fruit and vegetable consumption among students, supporting local farmers and rural communities, and providing nutrition and agriculture education to school districts and farmers. HHFKA amended existing child nutrition programs to establish mandatory funding of $5 million per year for competitive farm-to-school grants that support schools and nonprofit entities in establishing farm-to-school programs that improve a school's access to locally produced foods.[80]

---

[77] For the formula for administrative and oversight/monitoring costs, see Section 7 of the Child Nutrition Act of 1966 (codified at 42 U.S.C. 1776).

[78] See USDA-FNS website, http://www.fns.usda.gov/hussc/healthierus-school-challenge-smarter-lunchrooms.

[79] USDA, *The Farm to School Program—2012-2015: Four Years in Review*, p. 3. https://fns-prod.azureedge.net/sites/default/files/f2s/Farm-to-School-at-USDA—4-Years-in-Review.pdf.

[80] HHFKA, Section 243 (Access to Local Foods: Farm to School Program), amending §18 of the Richard B. Russell National School Lunch Act (42 U.S.C. 1758(j)). In addition, appropriations are authorized "such sums as are necessary for each of fiscal years 2011 through 2015."

The FY2018 appropriations law provided an additional $5 million in discretionary funding to remain available until expended.[81] Grants may be used for training, supporting operations, planning, purchasing equipment, developing school gardens, developing partnerships, and implementing farm-to-school programs. USDA's Office of Community Food Systems provides additional resources on farm-to-school issues.[82]

Through an Administrative Review process (formerly referred to as Coordinated Review Effort (CRE)), USDA-FNS, in cooperation with state agencies, conducts periodic on-site NSLP school compliance and accountability evaluations to improve management and identify administrative, subsidy claim, and meal quality problems.[83] State agencies are required to conduct administrative reviews of all school food authorities (SFAs) that operate the NSLP under their jurisdiction at least once during a three-year review cycle.[84] Federal Administrative Review expenditures were approximately $9.9 million in FY2017.

USDA-FNS and state agencies conduct many other child nutrition program support activities for which dedicated funding is provided. Among other examples, there is the Institute of Child Nutrition (ICN), which provides technical assistance, instruction, and materials related to nutrition and food service management; it receives $5 million a year in mandatory funding appropriated in statute. ICN is located at the University of Mississippi. USDA-FNS provides training on food safety education. Funding is also provided for USDA-FNS to conduct studies, provide training and technical assistance, and oversee payment accuracy.

---

[81] See Section 763 of P.L. 115-141.

[82] See USDA-FNS's Office of Community Food Systems: http://www.fns.usda.gov/farmtoschool/farm-school.

[83] Text in this paragraph is adapted from the USDA-FNS, *National School Lunch Program: Coordinated Review Effort (CRE)*, FNS-640 Data Report, January 2014.

[84] HHFKA increased the frequency of administrative reviews from once every five years to once every three years. See final rule at USDA Food and Nutrition Service, "Administrative Reviews in the School Nutrition Programs," 81 *Federal Register* 50170, July 29, 2016.

APPENDIX A. ACRONYMS USED IN THIS CHAPTER

Table A.1. Acronyms

Government Agencies	
USDA	U.S. Department of Agriculture
USDA-FNS	Food and Nutrition Service
Programs	
CACFP	Child and Adult Care Food Program
FFVP	Fresh Fruit and Vegetable Program
NSLP	National School Lunch Program
SBP	School Breakfast Program
SEBTC	Summer Electronic Benefits Transfer for Children
SFSP	Summer Food Service Program
SMP	Special Milk Program
Miscellaneous	
CEP	Community Eligibility Provision
CPI-U	Consumer Price Index for All Urban Consumers
FPL	Federal Poverty Level
HHFKA	Healthy, Hunger-Free Kids Act of 2010 (P.L. 111-296)
IOM	Institute of Medicine
LEA	Local Educational Agency
RCCI	Residential Child Care Institution
SFA	School Food Authority

APPENDIX B. PER-MEAL OR PER-SNACK REIMBURSEMENT RATES FOR CHILD NUTRITION PROGRAMS[85]

This appendix lists the specific reimbursement rates discussed in the earlier sections of the report. Reimbursement rates are adjusted for inflation for each school or calendar year according to terms laid out in the

[85] All reimbursement rate tables in this Appendix display rates for the 48 continental U.S. states. For Alaska, Hawaii, and territories where applicable, please see the source USDA-FNS *Federal Register* notice.

programs' authorizing laws. Each year, the new rates are announced in the *Federal Register*.[86]

Table B.I. Reimbursement Rates, NSLP: *Lunches* Per-meal reimbursements for 48 states and DC, school year 2018-2019

Meal Type	Serve Less than 60% of Lunches as Free and Reduced-Price	Serve 60% or More of Lunches as Free or Reduced-Price	Bonus Available for School Districts Certified as Compliant with Nutrition Guidelines
Free	$3.31	$3.33	+$0.06
Reduced-price	$2.91	$2.93	+$0.06
Paid	$0.31	$0.33	+$0.06

Source: USDA-FNS, https://www.federalregister.gov/documents/2018/07/19/2018-15465/national-school-lunchspecial-milk-and-school-breakfast-programs-national-average-paymentsmaximum. For NSLP reimbursement rates for other years, Alaska, Hawaii, and/or participating territories, see USDA-FNS website: https://www.fns.usda.gov/school-meals/rates-reimbursement.

Note: For school year 2018-2019, the maximum rate for 48 states and DC is $3.48 per free meal, $3.08 per reduced-price meal, and $0.30 per paid meal (and an additional $0.06 for nutrition guidelines). The maximum rate is the maximum per-lunch rate that a state can provide a school food authority.

Table B.2. Reimbursement Rates, NSLP: *After-School Snacks* Per-snack reimbursements for 48 states and DC, school year 2018-2019

Snack Type	Reimbursement
Free	$0.91
Reduced-price	$0.45
Paid	$0.08

Source: USDA-FNS. For after-school snack NSLP reimbursement rates for other years, Alaska, Hawaii, and/or participating territories, see USDA-FNS website: https://www.fns.usda.gov/school-meals/rates-reimbursement.

[86] For more detail on how inflation adjustment is conducted, see the child nutrition program sections of CRS Report R42000, *Inflation-Indexing Elements in Federal Entitlement Programs*, coordinated by Dawn Nuschler.

Table B.3. Reimbursement Rates, SBP Per-meal reimbursement for 48 states and DC, school year 2018-2019

Meal Type	Nonsevere Need (less than 40% free or reduced price)[a]	Severe Need (greater than or equal to 40% free or reduced price)[a]
Free	$1.79	$2.14
Reduced-price	$1.49	$1.84
Paid	$0.31	$0.31

Source: USDA-FNS. For NSLP reimbursement rates for other years, Alaska, Hawaii, and/or participating territories, see USDA-FNS website: https://www.fns.usda.gov/school-meals/rates-reimbursement.

[a.] Generally, severe need status is determined based on the percentage of meals served two school years prior to the year the currently reimbursed meal is served. For example, a school district's severe need status in school year 2018-2019 would be calculated based on meals served in school year 2016-2017.

Table B.4. Commodity Food Assistance, NSLP and CACFP (Centers) Rate per-meal for school year 2018-2019

	For Each NSLP/CACFP Meal Served
Commodity Food Reimbursement	$0.2350

Source: USDA, Food and Nutrition Service, "Food Distribution Program: Value of Donated Foods From July 1, 2018, Through June 30, 2019," 83 Federal Register 35607, July 1, 2018.

Notes: For past years, see USDA-FNS website: http://www.fns.usda.gov/fdd/value-donated-foods-notices. SFSP has a different commodity food assistance rate, see Table B.7.

Table B.5. Reimbursement Rates, CACFP: Child Care Centers, At-Risk After-School Programs Per-meal/snack reimbursement for 48 States and DC, school year 2018-2019

	Lunch/Supper	Breakfast	Snack
Free	$3.31	$1.79	$0.91
Reduced-price	$2.91	$1.49	$0.45
Paid	$0.31	$0.31	$0.08

Source: For historical program reimbursement rates as well as Alaska's and Hawaii's rates, see http://www.fns.usda.gov/cacfp/reimbursement-rates.

Notes: These reimbursement rates are identical to NSLP and SBP rates.

Table B.6. Reimbursement Rates, CACFP: *Child Care Homes* Per-meal/snack reimbursement for 48 States and DC, school year 2018-2019

	Lunch/Supper	**Breakfast**	**Snack**
Tier I	$2.46	$1.31	$0.73
Tier II	$1.48	$0.48	$0.20

Source: For historical program reimbursement rates as well as Alaska's and Hawaii's rates, see http://www.fns.usda.gov/cacfp/reimbursement-rates.

Note: CACFP also provides administrative reimbursements to sponsoring organizations of day care homes. Based on the number of homes sponsored, funding is provided per home, per month. These rates are not displayed in this table but are included in USDA, Food and Nutrition Service, "Child and Adult Care Food Program: National Average Payment Rates, Day Care Home Food Service Payment Rates, and Administrative Reimbursement Rates for Sponsoring Organizations of Day Care Homes for the Period July 1, 2018 Through June 30, 2019," 83 Federal Register 34108, July 1, 2018.

Table B.7. Reimbursement Rates, SFSP Per-meal/snack reimbursement for 48 states and DC (rounded to nearest cent), calendar year 2018

	Lunch/Supper		**Breakfast**		**Snack**	
	Rural or Self-Prep	All Other Sites	Rural or Self-Prep	All Other Sites	Rural or Self-Prep	All Other Sites
Operating	$3.55	$3.55	$2.03	$2.03	$0.83	$0.83
Component						
Administrative	$0.37	$0.31	$0.20	$0.16	$0.10	$0.08
Component						
Combined (Total)	$3.92	$3.86	$2.23	$2.19	$0.93	$0.91
Rate						

Source: For program reimbursement rates as well as Alaska's and Hawaii's rates, see USDA, Food and Nutrition Service, "Summer Food Service Program; 2018 Reimbursement Rates," 83 Federal Register 4025, January 29, 2018.

Note: Per authorizing law, the administrative component is calculated to the nearest quarter-cent. This table rounds to the nearest cent. As the table shows, the administrative component varies slightly (e.g., by about 5 cents for lunches) depending on the location of the site (e.g., rural vs. urban) and whether meals are prepared on-site or by a vendor. For meals prepared on-site, providers receive 1.5 cents per meal in USDA commodity foods.

Table B.8. Reimbursement Rates, SMP Per half-pint reimbursement for 48 States and DC (rounded to nearest cent), school year 2018-2019

	All Milk Served	Paid Milk	Free Milk to Low Income Children
Schools that only sell milk	$0.21	Not applicable	Not applicable
Schools that sell and provide free milk	Not applicable	$0.21	Average cost per half-pint of milk
Schools that provide only free milk	$0.21	Not applicable	Not applicable

Source: For program reimbursement rates, see https://www.fns.usda.gov/school-meals/rates-reimbursement.

In: Child Nutrition Programs
Editor: Daniel D. Coleman
ISBN: 978-1-53615-764-2

Chapter 4

SUMMER MEALS: ACTIONS NEEDED TO IMPROVE PARTICIPATION ESTIMATES AND ADDRESS PROGRAM CHALLENGES*

United States Government Accountability Office

ABBREVIATIONS

ADA	average daily attendance
CACFP	Child and Adult Care Food Program
EBT	Electronic Benefits Transfer
eSFSP	Enhanced Summer Food Service Program
FNS	Food and Nutrition Service
NSLP	National School Lunch Program
SBP	School Breakfast Program
SFSP	Summer Food Service Program
SNAP	Supplemental Nutrition Assistance Program

* This is an edited, reformatted and augmented version of United States Government Accountability Office; Report to Congressional Requesters, Publication No. GAO-18-369, dated May 2018.

Summer EBT	Summer Electronic Benefit Transfer for Children
USDA	U.S. Department of Agriculture
WIC	Special Supplemental Nutrition Program for Women, Infants, and Children

WHY GAO DID THIS STUDY

The SFSP, a federal nutrition assistance program, is intended to provide food to children in low-income areas during periods when area schools are closed for vacation. In the last decade, federal expenditures for SFSP have increased as the program has expanded, according to USDA data. GAO was asked to review the SFSP.

This chapter examines (1) what is known about SFSP participation, (2) other programs that help feed low-income children over the summer, and (3) challenges, if any, in providing summer meals to children and the extent to which USDA provides assistance to address these challenges. GAO reviewed relevant federal laws, regulations, and guidance; analyzed USDA's SFSP data for fiscal years 2007 through 2016; surveyed state agencies responsible for administering the SFSP in 50 states and the District of Columbia; visited a nongeneralizable group of 3 states and 30 meal sites, selected based on Census data on child poverty rates and urban and rural locations; analyzed meal site data from the 3 states; and interviewed USDA, state and national organization officials, and SFSP providers, including sponsors and site operators.

WHAT GAO RECOMMENDS

GAO is making four recommendations, including that USDA improve estimates of children's participation in SFSP and communicate the circumstances it considers when granting flexibilities to ensure safe meal delivery. USDA generally agreed with GAO's recommendations.

What GAO Found

Nationwide, the total number of meals served to children in low-income areas through the Summer Food Service Program (SFSP) increased from 113 to 149 million (about 32 percent) from fiscal year 2007 through 2016. The U.S. Department of Agriculture (USDA) directs states to use the number of meals served, along with other data, to estimate the number of children participating in the SFSP. However, participation estimates have been calculated inconsistently from state to state and year to year. In 2017, USDA took steps to improve the consistency of participation estimates, noting they are critical for informing program implementation and strategic planning. However, GAO determined that the method USDA directs states to use will continue to provide unreliable estimates of participation, hindering USDA's ability to use them for these purposes.

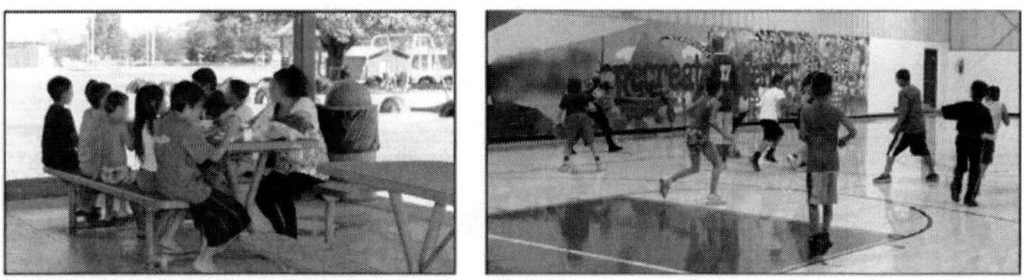

Source: GAO. | GAO-18-369.

Other federal and nonfederal programs help feed low-income children over the summer to some extent, according to states GAO surveyed and SFSP providers and others GAO interviewed. For example, in July 2016, USDA data indicate about 26 million meals were served through a separate federal program that allows school meal providers to serve summer meals. Some children also received summer meals through nonfederal programs operated by faith-based organizations and foodbanks, though GAO's state survey and interviews with providers and national organizations indicate the reach of such efforts is limited.

States and SFSP providers reported challenges with meal sites, participation, and program administration; USDA has taken steps to address these areas. Specifically, in GAO's survey, a majority of states reported challenges with availability and awareness of meal sites, as well as limited program participation and administrative capacity. National, state, and local officials have taken steps to address these issues, such as increasing outreach and offering activities to attract participation. In addition, 17 states in GAO's survey and providers in the states GAO visited reported a challenge with ensuring meal sites are in safe locations. To address this safety issue, USDA has granted some states and sponsors flexibility from the requirement that children consume meals on-site. However, USDA has not broadly communicated the circumstances it considers when granting this flexibility. Further, some states and sponsors that have requested this flexibility reported difficulty obtaining data to show these circumstances exist, hampering their ability to ensure safe meal delivery.

May 31, 2018

The Honorable Virginia Foxx
Chairwoman
Committee on Education and the Workforce
House of Representatives

The Honorable Todd Rokita Chairman
Subcommittee on Early Childhood, Elementary and Secondary Education
House of Representatives

In fiscal year 2016, the U.S. Department of Agriculture (USDA) spent $478 million to provide more than 150 million meals to children through the Summer Food Service Program (SFSP). As a federal nutrition assistance program, the primary purpose of the SFSP is to provide food service to children in low-income areas during periods when area schools are closed for vacation. USDA's Food and Nutrition Service (FNS) oversees the SFSP, which is administered by the states and operated by a variety of public and private nonprofit organizations and government entities that sponsor meals at sites such as schools, camps, parks, churches, and libraries. In the last decade, federal expenditures have increased as the program has expanded, according to FNS data. As Congress considers proposals intended to modify child nutrition programs, you asked that we examine issues related to the SFSP.

This chapter assesses:

1) What is known about participation in the Summer Food Service Program and how it has changed in the last 10 years?
2) What other programs help feed low-income children over the summer?
3) What challenges exist, if any, in providing summer meals to children, and to what extent does FNS provide assistance to states and sponsors to address these challenges?

To address our first objective about participation in the SFSP, we analyzed FNS's national data on SFSP meals served for fiscal years 2007 through 2016. For context on these trends, we analyzed, and compared to the SFSP data, FNS's data on lunches served through the National School Lunch Program (NSLP), the largest child nutrition assistance program, for the same time period. To assess the reliability of SFSP and NSLP data, we (1) performed electronic testing of relevant data elements, (2) reviewed existing information about the data and the system that produced them, and (3) interviewed agency officials knowledgeable about the data. We determined that these data were sufficiently reliable to identify the number of meals served in each program and assess change over time.

We also reviewed FNS's method for estimating the number of children participating in the SFSP using these data and discuss the reliability of this method in the body of the report. From our three selected states, we also analyzed site-level data on meals served and days of operation for 2 months during the summer of 2016, including the month with the largest number of SFSP meals served in each state. We assessed the reliability of these data by (1) performing electronic testing of relevant data elements,

(2) reviewing existing information about the data and the system that produced them, and (3) interviewing agency officials knowledgeable about the data. We determined these data to be sufficiently reliable for the purposes of this chapter.

To obtain information specific to our second objective on other programs that help feed children in the summer, we also analyzed FNS data on meals served through the NSLP and School Breakfast Program (SBP) in July 2016 because FNS used these data to estimate meals served through the Seamless Summer Option in summer 2016.[1] To assess the reliability of these data, we (1) performed electronic testing of relevant data elements, (2) reviewed existing information about the data and the system that produced them, and (3) interviewed agency officials knowledgeable about the data. We determined that these data were sufficiently reliable to describe the number of meals served through the Seamless Summer Option.

In addition, we relied on several methods to address all three objectives. At the federal level, we reviewed relevant federal laws, regulations, and guidance, and interviewed FNS officials in headquarters and its seven regional offices. We also surveyed the state agencies responsible for administering the SFSP in the 50 states and District of Columbia. We administered our web-based survey between August and October 2017 and received a 100 percent response rate. Further, we visited three selected states—Arizona, Illinois, and Massachusetts—between June and July 2017. In each state, we interviewed state agency officials responsible for administering the SFSP, as well as selected SFSP providers, and we observed SFSP meal service at a total of 30 meal sites.[2] We selected states and local areas within those states based on a high proportion of children in poverty, a mix of urban and rural densities, a mix

[1] States report monthly to FNS the number of meals served through the NSLP and SBP using the FNS-10 form. The information reported for the NSLP and SBP includes the number of paid, free, and reduced-price meals by meal type (e.g., lunches and breakfasts) for each month. FNS's estimate of the number of meals served through the Seamless Summer Option over the summer includes free and reduced-price lunches and snacks served through the NSLP and free and reduced-price breakfasts served through the SBP in July in all states.

[2] Throughout our report, references to "SFSP providers" include both sponsors of SFSP sites and meal site operators, if different from the sponsor.

of sponsor and site types, and diverse locations in the country. We visited a wide variety of site locations including, but not limited to, schools, parks, community recreation areas, and libraries. To gather additional information, we interviewed a broad range of regional and national organizations involved in the SFSP, such as the Boys and Girls Club of America, Catholic Charities, and Feeding America. Additional information on the report's scope and methodology is included in appendix I.

We conducted this work from January 2017 through May 2018 in accordance with generally accepted government auditing standards. Those standards require that we plan and perform the audit to obtain sufficient, appropriate evidence to provide a reasonable basis for our findings and conclusions based on our audit objectives. We believe that the evidence obtained provides a reasonable basis for our findings and conclusions based on our audit objectives.

BACKGROUND

Created in 1968, the SFSP is authorized under the Richard B. Russell National School Lunch Act and generally provides free meals to children age 18 and under in low-income areas during certain periods when school is not in session.[3] Specifically, the SFSP operates during school summer vacation periods between May through September, vacation periods in any month for programs operating on a continuous school calendar, and certain other times for areas affected by an unanticipated school closure, such as for a natural disaster. However, the majority of SFSP meals are served to children during the summer months.

[3] Codified as amended at 42 U.S.C. § 1761. Eligible children also include individuals over age 18 who are determined by a state educational agency or a local public educational agency of a state to have a disability, and who are participating in a public or nonprofit private school program established for individuals who have a disability.

In fiscal years 2007 through 2016, federal expenditures on SFSP increased, according to FNS data, though there was a slight decrease between fiscal years 2015 and 2016 (see Figure 1).[4]

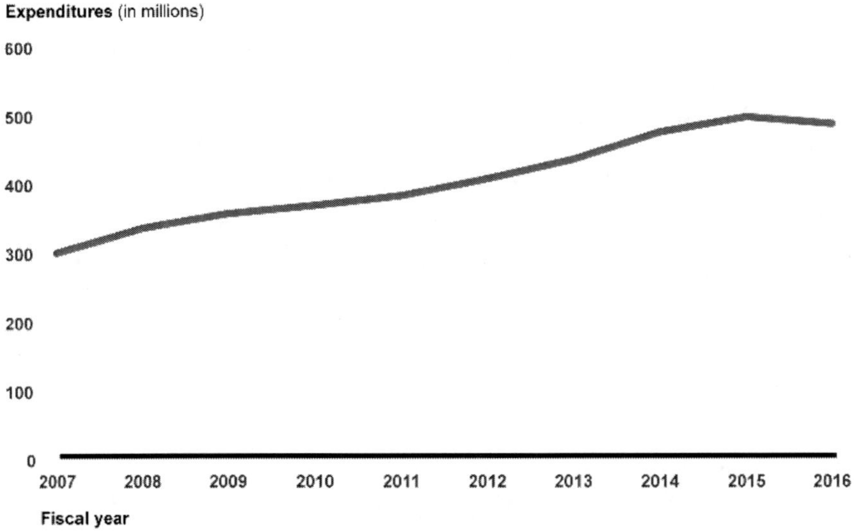

Source: GAO analysis of Food and Nutrition Service data. | GAO-18-369.

Note: This figure includes federal expenditures such as cash payments for meals served; state and sponsor administrative costs; and health inspection costs.

Figure 1. Summer Food Service Program Federal Expenditures, Fiscal Years 2007 through 2016.

SFSP Program Administration

The SFSP is administered at the federal level by FNS through its national and regional offices. FNS is responsible for issuing regulations,[5] instructions, and guidance; reviewing states' program management and administration plans; overseeing program administration; and reimbursing

[4] As of April 2018, preliminary fiscal year 2017 expenditures totaled $483 million dollars, which are similar to fiscal year 2016 expenditures.

[5] The SFSP program regulations are found at 7 C.F.R. pt. 225.

states for meals served that meet program requirements.[6] At the state level, the program is administered by state agencies and locally operated by state-approved sponsors, such as school districts, local government entities, or private nonprofit organizations.[7] State agencies are responsible for approving, providing training to, and inspecting and monitoring sponsors and meal sites. Sponsors, in turn, are responsible for monitoring their SFSP meal sites, managing the meal service, and providing training to administrative staff and site operators. A sponsor may operate one site or multiple sites.[8] Sites are physical locations in the community where children receive and consume meals in a supervised setting. According to FNS guidance, sites may be located in a variety of settings, including schools, parks, community centers, health clinics, hospitals, apartment complexes, churches, and migrant camps.

SFSP Program Requirements

States may approve different types of SFSP meal sites, including open sites, closed enrolled sites, and camps. Open sites operate in an area where at least half of the children are eligible for free or reduced-price school meals (referred to as "area eligible"), according to data from entities such as schools or the U.S. Census Bureau. Children are generally eligible for free or reduced-price school meals if their households have incomes at or below 185 percent of federal poverty guidelines.[9] At open sites, meals are

---

6 States, in turn, provide funds to sponsors. Federal funding is also provided for certain SFSP administrative and operating costs.

7 The type of state agency responsible for administering the SFSP depends on the state and could include the state educational, health, social services, or agriculture agency. Depending on the state, the state agency administering the SFSP may or may not be the same agency that oversees other child nutrition programs.

8 In our report, we use the term "sponsor" when referring to entities operating SFSP sites. A sponsor may be approved to operate a maximum of 200 sites and serve a maximum total average daily attendance of 50,000 children. Exceptions to these limits may be approved by the state agency if the sponsor can demonstrate that it has the capability to manage a larger program.

9 The federal poverty guidelines are derived from the poverty thresholds that the Census Bureau uses to prepare its estimates of the number of individuals and families in poverty, based on household size and income. The guidelines are updated annually by the Department of

made available to all children in the area, and all meals served that meet program requirements are reimbursable. Closed enrolled sites, on the other hand, are open only to enrolled children, as opposed to the community at large. At closed enrolled sites, meals served to all children in attendance are reimbursable as long as at least half of the enrolled children are eligible for free or reduced-price school lunch.[10] Unlike other types of sites, camps are reimbursed only for meals served to children who have been individually determined to be eligible for free or reduced-price school meals.

SFSP meals must meet certain requirements in order to be eligible for federal reimbursement; for example, the meals must be served and consumed on-site at an approved site.[11] Federal reimbursements for summer meals are provided for each breakfast, lunch, supper, or snack served to an eligible child at an eligible site that also meets federal requirements for menu components, scheduled meal times, and nutrition.[12] For example, to meet nutritional requirements, a lunch or a supper must, at a minimum, include four components: 2 ounces of meat or a comparable serving of a meat alternate, 3/4 cup of fruits and/or vegetables (at least two kinds), a slice of bread or a comparable serving of another grain, and a cup of milk.[13] In 2017, the federal reimbursement rate was $3.83 or $3.77 for

---

Health and Human Services, adjusting for inflation, and are used to determine eligibility for certain federal programs and benefits. Using the federal poverty guidelines, FNS annually publishes income eligibility guidelines for determining eligibility for free and reduced price meals. For July 1, 2017 through June 30, 2018, 185 percent of the federal poverty guidelines for a family of four in the contiguous 48 states and D.C. was an annual income of $45,510. See Child Nutrition Programs: Income Eligibility Guidelines, 82 Fed. Reg. 17,182 (Apr. 10, 2017).

[10] Eligibility for closed enrolled sites may be determined through applications completed by household members on behalf of the child enrolled or other sources of information that can be used to determine site eligibility, such as school or census data.

[11] Specifically, program regulations require sponsors to maintain children on site while meals are consumed. 7 C.F.R. § 225.6(e)(15). This requirement, sometimes referred to as the "congregate meal requirement," is referred to as the "on-site requirement" throughout the report. In general, only meals served to children may be claimed as reimbursable meals. However, in certain circumstances, meals served to adults may be counted as operating costs.

[12] See 7 C.F.R. § 225.16.

[13] In comparison, lunches served in the NSLP must include five components – meat or meat alternate, fruits, vegetables, grains, and milk. NSLP lunches must also meet additional

each eligible SFSP lunch or supper served, depending on the type of meal site.[14] Each site may serve up to two meals or one meal and one snack per day.[15]

Some flexibilities are available to FNS in implementing the SFSP program, under its waiver and demonstration authorities. Specifically, the National School Lunch Act authorizes the Secretary of Agriculture to waive, upon request of a state or eligible service provider, certain program requirements established under the National School Lunch Act or the Child Nutrition Act of 1966, as amended, including some for the SFSP.[16] In order to grant a waiver request, the Secretary must determine that the waiver would facilitate the state or service provider's ability to carry out the purpose of the program, and that the waiver will not increase the overall cost of the program to the federal government, among other things.[17] In the event a waiver request is submitted, the Secretary is required to act promptly and state in writing whether the waiver request is granted or denied, and why. The Secretary is also required to periodically review the performance of waiver recipients, and submit an annual report to Congress summarizing the use of waivers and their effectiveness, among other details.[18]

---

requirements, such as calorie maximums that vary by student grade groups, which SFSP lunches do not have to meet.

[14] Specifically, in 2017, the lunch or supper reimbursement rate for rural sites and those sites that prepare the meals themselves was $3.83 and $3.77 per meal for all other types of meal sites in all states except for Alaska and Hawaii. The reimbursement rates for breakfast were $2.19 and $2.15 per meal, and for snacks were $0.91 and $0.89 per meal. Reimbursement rates are annually adjusted.

[15] However, sites generally cannot serve both lunch and supper on the same day. Some exceptions apply: for example, camps and sites that primarily serve children from migrant families may be approved to serve up to three meals or two meals and one snack each day.

[16] 42 U.S.C. § 1760(l). Eligible service providers include SFSP sponsors. This waiver authority is subject to specified exceptions; for example, the Secretary may not grant waivers that relate to the nutritional content of meals served or federal reimbursement rates, among other things.

[17] The statute requires waiver applications to describe 1) the statutory or regulatory requirements that are requested to be waived; 2) in the case of a state, the actions, if any, that the state has undertaken to remove state statutory or regulatory barriers; 3) the goal of the waiver to improve services under the program and expected outcomes; and 4) the impediments to the efficient operation and administration of the program.

[18] Specifically, the Secretary is required to annually submit to the Committee on Education and Labor of the House of Representatives and the Committee on Agriculture, Nutrition, and Forestry of the Senate a report that summarizes the use of waivers by the state and eligible

In addition to this waiver authority, the Secretary is also authorized to carry out demonstration projects to develop and test methods of providing access to summer meals for low-income children in urban and rural areas, to reduce or eliminate the food insecurity and hunger of low-income children and improve their nutritional status.[19] The Secretary is required to provide for an independent evaluation of the demonstration projects carried out under this authority, and submit an annual report to Congress on the status of each project and the results of the evaluations.[20]

NUMBER OF SFSP MEALS SERVED HAS GENERALLY INCREASED SINCE 2007, BUT ESTIMATES OF CHILDREN PARTICIPATING IN THE SFSP ARE UNRELIABLE

Number of SFSP Meals Served Has Increased by 32 Percent since Fiscal Year 2007

The total number of SFSP meals served nationwide during the summer— one indicator of program participation—increased from 113 million meals in fiscal year 2007 to 149 million meals in fiscal year 2016,

service providers; describes whether the waivers resulted in improved services to children; describes the impact of the waivers on providing nutritional meals to participants; and describes how the waivers reduced the quantity of paperwork necessary to administer the program.

[19] This demonstration authority was first established and funded by the Agriculture, Rural Development, Food and Drug Administration, and Related Agencies Appropriations Act, 2010, Pub. L. No. 111-80, § 749(g), 123 Stat. 2090, 2132-33. Subsequent appropriations acts continued to fund these demonstrations, most recently the Consolidated Appropriations Act, 2018, Pub. L. No. 115-141, div. A, tit. IV, 132 Stat. 348.

[20] Specifically, each December 31, the Secretary is required to submit a report to the Committee on Education and Labor of the House of Representatives and the Committee on Agriculture, Nutrition, and Forestry of the Senate a report that includes the status of each demonstration project and the results of the evaluations for the previous fiscal year. Further, not later than 120 days after the completion of the last evaluation, the Secretary is required to submit a report to the same committees that includes recommendations to improve children's access to food during the summer months when school is not in regular session.

or by 32 percent, according to our analysis of FNS data.[21] The number of SFSP meals served has generally increased from year to year over this 10-year period. Most recently, meals decreased by 6 percent from 156 million meals in summer 2015 to 149 million meals in summer 2016, according to our analysis of FNS data (see Figure 2).[22] Factors that may have affected year-to-year fluctuations include changes in funding for summer programs, sponsor participation, weather, and the number of weekdays available for sites to serve meals within a given summer, according to FNS and state agency officials we interviewed. For example, state agency officials in one of the three selected states we visited said they believe that reductions in state and local funding for summer programs that also provide meals, and turnover of sponsors, including losing one of the state's largest sponsors in a recent summer, affected the total number of SFSP meals served in their state in 2016.

According to our analysis of FNS data, SFSP lunches served in the summer months increased by over 17 million from fiscal year 2007 through fiscal year 2016, accounting for almost half of the total increase in the number of SFSP meals served in that period.[23] However, when comparing across each of the meal types, supper and breakfast had the largest percentage increases over the 10-year period, 50 and 48 percent, respectively (see Table 1).[24] In comparison, the number of SFSP lunches

---

[21] Unless otherwise noted, this chapter focuses on SFSP meals served during the summer months, which we define to include May, June, July, and August, and nationwide refers to the 50 states and the District of Columbia. The SFSP operates during school vacation from May through September, during vacation periods in any month for programs operating on continuous school calendars, and during certain other times for areas affected by unanticipated school closure, such as for a natural disaster. While meals are served under the SFSP throughout the year, the majority of meals are served to children during the summer months. For example, in fiscal year 2016, meals served during summer months accounted for more than 99 percent of all SFSP meals. In addition, our review focused on fiscal year 2007 through fiscal year 2016, and included all meals served: breakfast, lunch, supper, and snack.

[22] As of April 2018, preliminary data for fiscal year 2017 indicate 148 million SFSP meals were served in the summer months, continuing the decrease from fiscal year 2015.

[23] Our analyses of SFSP meals in this chapter include SFSP meals served during the summer months—which we define to include May, June, July, and August.

[24] When looking at the overall decline in SFSP meals served from fiscal year 2015 to fiscal year 2016, snacks had the largest percentage decrease at 9 percent, or 1.4 million meals, while breakfast, lunch, and supper each declined by between 2 and 4 percent.

served increased by 26 percent from fiscal years 2007 through fiscal year 2016.

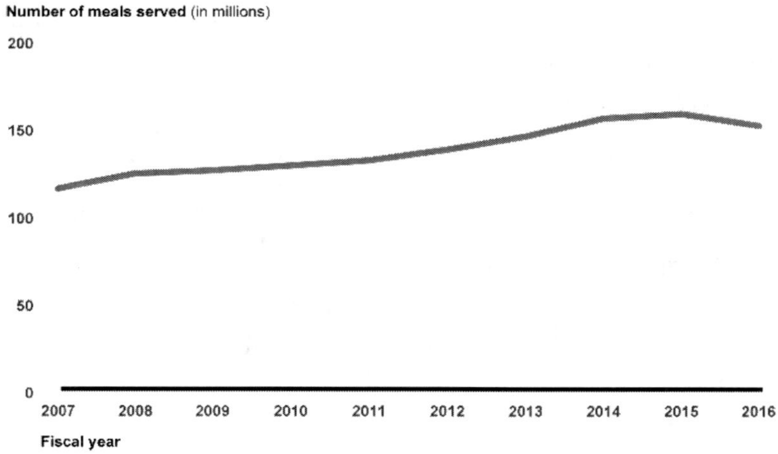

Source: GAO analysis of Food and Nutrition Service data. | GAO-18-369.

Note: SFSP meals served include breakfast, lunch, supper, and snack. This figure includes meals served in the 50 states and District of Columbia during May, June, July, and August.

Figure 2. Number of Summer Food Service Program (SFSP) Meals Served Nationwide during the Summer, Fiscal Years 2007 through 2016.

Table 1. Change in Number of Meals Served Nationwide in the Food and Nutrition Service's Summer Food Service Program (SFSP) by Meal Type, Fiscal Years 2007 and 2016

	Number of SFSP Meals Served by Meal Service Type				
Fiscal year	Breakfast	Lunch	Supper	Snack	Total
2007	28,512,170	68,085,416	4,166,516	12,210,737	112,974,839
2016	42,329,229	85,708,601	6,254,579	14,868,097	149,160,506
Increase in number of meals served	13,817,059	17,623,185	2,088,063	2,657,360	36,185,667
Percent increase	48%	26%	50%	22%	n/a

Legend: n/a = not applicable.

Source: GAO analysis of data provided by the Food and Nutrition Service. I GAO-18-369.

Note: SFSP meals served include breakfast, lunch, supper, and snack. This figure includes meals served in the 50 states and District of Columbia during May, June, July, and August. Our review focused on changes in the 10 years from fiscal year 2007 through fiscal year 2016.

From fiscal year 2007 through fiscal year 2016, there were increases in the numbers of meals served in both SFSP and NSLP, the largest child nutrition assistance program. Specifically, SFSP lunches served in July increased from 32 million to 40 million, or 24 percent, from fiscal year 2007 to 2016, and NSLP lunches served in March increased from 328 million to 376 million meals, or 15 percent, according to our analysis of FNS data.[25] Although the programs generally serve similar populations, different factors likely affected the number of meals served by each program, in part because NSLP serves children in schools during the school year and SFSP serves children in a variety of settings during the summer months.[26]

Estimates of Children Participating in SFSP Have Been Calculated Inconsistently and Are Unreliable

Although states report the actual number of SFSP meals served to FNS, they *estimate* the number of children participating in SFSP, and information obtained from our state survey and FNS indicate that these participation estimates have been calculated inconsistently.[27] FNS instructs state agencies on how to calculate a statewide estimate of children's participation in the SFSP, referred to as average daily attendance (ADA), using sponsor-reported information on the number of meals served and

---

[25] We compared the month that each program served the most meals which, according to FNS officials, is July for SFSP and March for NSLP. As of April 2018, preliminary fiscal year 2017 data indicate that 403 million NSLP lunches were served in March and 39 million SFSP lunches were served in July, representing an increase in the number of NSLP lunches served, but a slight decline in the number of SFSP lunches served, compared to the prior year.

[26] For more information on recent trends in the number of NSLP meals served see GAO, *School Nutrition: USDA Has Efforts Underway to Help Address Ongoing Challenges Implementing Changes in Nutrition Standards*, GAO-15-656 (Washington, D.C.: Sept. 14, 2015) and GAO, *School Lunch: Implementing Nutritional Changes Was Challenging and Clarification of Oversight Requirements is Needed*, GAO-14-104 (Washington, D.C.: Jan. 28, 2014).

[27] For reimbursement purposes, states are required to report monthly data on the number of SFSP meals served. Once a year, FNS requires states to use these data to estimate program participation; however, this estimate is not used for reimbursement purposes.

days of operation in July of each year.[28] However, states' methods for calculating ADA have differed from state to state and from year to year, according to our review of states' survey responses and FNS documents. For example, although FNS directed states to include the number of meals served in each site's primary meal service— which may or may not be lunch—some states, according to our survey and FNS data, were calculating ADA using only meals served at lunch. FNS officials told us that these states were therefore not following the agency's instructions. Further, some states have changed their methods for calculating ADA over time—five states reported in our survey that the method they used to calculate ADA in fiscal year 2016 differed from the one they used previously.[29]

Excerpt from Food and Nutrition Service's Revised Average Daily Attendance (ADA) Calculation Instructions for the Summer Food Service Program (SFSP)

"ADA is calculated by taking the total number of meals served in each site's primary meal service during the claim period and dividing that number by the number of operating or meal service days for the site during that claim period. A site's primary meal service is the meal at which the most meals are claimed. For most sites, this is typically lunch; however, if a site serves more meals at breakfast than at lunch, then breakfast would be considered the primary meal service. Once the ADA is calculated for each site, the sponsor will then add the ADAs for all sites that the sponsor manages. This will result in the ADA for the sponsor....Each site's primary meal service must be used in the Total ADA calculation for the sponsor [and then] this number should be added to the Total ADA for all other sponsors to get the cumulative ADA of Sponsors that is entered on this form."

Source: FNS Form 418. | GAO-18-369.

---

[28] States report this information to FNS on Form FNS-418: Report of the Summer Food Service Program for Children. Sponsors first report to states a total ADA across all their sites, which is calculated by dividing the number of meals served at each site's primary meal service by the number of days each site operated in July, the month FNS has determined most SFSP meals are served, according to FNS officials. States combine sponsor ADAs for a statewide ADA for July. FNS combines states' estimates to estimate children's participation in the SFSP nationwide.

[29] Seven additional states reported that they were unsure if they had changed the method used to calculate ADA in fiscal year 2016.

While FNS clarified its instructions in May 2017 to help improve the consistency of states' ADA calculations moving forward, ADA remains an unreliable estimate of children's daily participation in SFSP for at least two reasons, according to our analysis. (See sidebar for the revised ADA calculation instructions.) First, ADA is based on summary data that does not account for existing variation in site days of operation, and second, it is based on July data, which does not reflect the month with the greatest number of meals served in every state.

- According to our analysis, ADA is an unreliable estimate of children's participation in SFSP because it currently does not account for existing variation in the number of days that each site serves meals to children. Specifically, because FNS's instructions indicate that sites' ADAs are to be combined to provide a statewide ADA estimate, differences in the number of days of meal service are disregarded. As a result, ADA does not reflect the average number of children served SFSP meals daily throughout the month. Our analysis of site-level data from one of the selected states illustrates this limitation. In this state, multiple sites reported an ADA of 60 for July, yet two of those sites served meals to children on only 1 day of the month and another site served meals to children on 20 days.[30] Although 120 children were served SFSP meals only 1 day in July across two of these sites, the combined ADA across all three sites, which we calculated following FNS's instructions, inaccurately suggests an average of 180 children were participating in SFSP at these sites on a daily basis in July.
- According to our analysis, ADA is also an unreliable estimate of children's participation in SFSP because it currently does not account for state variation in the month with the greatest number of SFSP meals served, potentially leading to an underestimate. According to FNS officials, the agency instructs states to calculate

---

[30] According to officials from some national organizations involved in the SFSP, meal sites operating for 1 day may be one-time events. Such one-time or special events could include a summer kick-off event in the community to help promote awareness of the program.

ADA for July because officials identified this as the month with the largest number of meals served nationwide. However, because of reasons such as state variations in school calendars, July is not the month with the largest number of meals served in every state. In one of the selected states, Arizona, using July to calculate ADA cuts the estimate almost in half.[31] Specifically, we followed FNS's instructions and calculated that Arizona's ADA was 14,987 in July 2016 compared to 26,772 in June 2016. Nationwide, in summer 2016, 26 states served more SFSP meals in June or August than in July, according to our analysis of FNS data. However, without site level data on meals served and operating days, the extent to which these states had higher ADAs in June or August as compared to July is unknown.

In its May 2017 memo to states revising the ADA calculation instructions, FNS said that it is critical that the agency's means of estimating children's participation in the SFSP is as accurate as possible because it helps inform program implementation at the national level and facilitates strategic planning and outreach to areas with low participation.[32] In addition, *Standards for Internal Control in the Federal Government* state that agencies should maintain quality data and process it into quality information that is shared with stakeholders to help achieve agency goals.[33]

Although FNS has also collected information on other data that states collect on the SFSP, the agency has not yet used this information to help improve its estimate of children's participation in the program.

---

[31] State agency officials and sponsors we spoke with in Arizona explained that schools typically end the academic year in May, with some schools returning to session in July and, therefore, June is the busiest month for SFSP in Arizona. On the other hand, officials in Illinois and Massachusetts told us that the SFSP usually serves the most meals in July because the academic year in those states typically ends in late June.

[32] USDA, Food and Nutrition Service, *Revisions to Instructions for the Calculation for Average Daily Attendance on the Form FNS-418*, Memo code SFSP 09-2017 (Alexandria, VA: May 10, 2017).

[33] GAO, *Standards for Internal Control in the Federal Government*, GAO-14-704G (Washington, D.C.: Sept. 10, 2014).

In 2015, FNS published a Request for Information, asking whether states or sponsors collect any SFSP data that are not reported to FNS.[34] While FNS received responses from only 15 states, these responses suggest that some states collect additional data, such as site-level data that may allow for an improved estimate of children's SFSP participation, potentially addressing the issues we found in our analysis. In response to the information FNS received, they followed up with up to 9 of the 15 states in 2016 and 2017 to explore the feasibility of collecting additional data and improving estimates of children's participation. Although they took these steps, FNS officials told us they are cognizant of the burden on states and site operators that would be associated with additional reporting requirements.[35] At this time, the agency has not taken further action to improve the estimate, such as addressing the reliability issues caused by variation in the number of operating days of meal sites and in the months with the greatest number of meals served by state. As a result, FNS's understanding of children's participation in the SFSP remains limited, which impairs its ability to both inform program implementation and facilitate strategic planning and outreach to areas with low participation.

[34] Request for Information: Summer Meal Programs Data Reporting Requirements, 80 Fed. Reg. 12,423 (Mar. 9, 2015). At that time, 5 of the 15 state agencies that responded indicated that they collected additional data beyond what is reported to FNS, according to FNS data collected through the Request for Information. In addition, 44 states reported in our survey that they collected SFSP site-level data beyond what is required by FNS. However, we did not collect information on the types of site-level data collected by states or how easily they could share such information with FNS.

[35] FNS officials indicated they are currently conducting a study related to child nutrition program reporting requirements, as required by the Consolidated Appropriations Act, 2017. The act provided funds for an independent study to identify the best means of consolidating and coordinating reporting requirements under child nutrition programs to eliminate redundancy, increase efficiency, and reduce the reporting burden on school food authorities and state agencies. Pub. L. No. 115-31, div. A, tit. I, 131 Stat. 135, 161. FNS officials said they expect the study to be completed in November 2018. They noted that some states expressed concerns in the ongoing study about the burden of child nutrition reporting requirements. Further, FNS officials noted that collection of additional information from states would require OMB approval under the Paperwork Reduction Act, and may also require regulatory changes.

Other Federal and Nonfederal Programs Help Feed Low-Income Children over the Summer to Some Extent

Other Federal Programs Provide Meals and Nutrition Assistance Benefits over the Summer

Other federal programs that operate solely in the summer, as well as those operating year-round, help feed low-income children in the summer months. These programs include the NSLP Seamless Summer Option, which provides nutrition assistance benefits solely in the summer, and several federal programs that operate year-round.

In July 2016, in addition to the 70 million meals provided through the SFSP, 26 million meals were provided to low-income children through school food authorities participating in the NSLP's Seamless Summer Option, according to FNS data.[36] The Seamless Summer Option was established in 2004, and according to FNS, streamlines administrative requirements to encourage school food authorities providing free or reduced-price meals during the school year under the NSLP and SBP to continue providing meals to low-income children when school is not in

[36] These data include meals provided in the 50 states and the District of Columbia. FNS's estimate of the number of meals served through the Seamless Summer Option over the summer includes the number of free and reduced-price lunches and snacks served through the NSLP and free and reduced-price breakfasts served through the SBP in July in all states. School food authorities may continue providing free and reduced-price meals to children enrolled in accredited academic summer school programs through the NSLP and SBP. FNS officials told us they do not know how many summer meals are provided through the Seamless Summer Option, specifically because the Seamless Summer Option and NSLP meals are combined when reported by states for reimbursement purposes. Although FNS does not know the actual number of meals served through the Seamless Summer Option, agency officials told us they believe the number of summer meals provided through the NSLP is small relative to the number of meals served through the Seamless Summer Option during the summer months. They noted that their use of July NSLP data to estimate the number of Seamless Summer Option meals has several limitations, including that it overestimates the number of meals served through the program for July and underestimates the number of meals served through the program for the entire summer.

session.[37] For example, officials from a national organization involved in summer meals told us the Seamless Summer Option makes it easier for school food authorities to provide summer meals because they continue working with the same state agency, reporting the same information to the state, and operating without having to transition to a separate program. Nonetheless, school food authorities can choose to provide free summer meals to children through either the SFSP or Seamless Summer Option,[38] and the majority of states (34) reported in our survey that a greater proportion of school food authorities participated in the SFSP than the Seamless Summer Option in summer 2016.[39] According to FNS and selected state officials, this may be related to the generally lower meal reimbursement rates school food authorities participating in the Seamless Summer Option receive compared to the rates received by those participating in the SFSP.[40]

---

[37] The Seamless Summer Option was established by the Child Nutrition and WIC Reauthorization Act of 2004, Pub. L. No. 108-265, § 116, 118 Stat. 729, 748 (codified at 42 U.S.C. § 1761(a)(8) and (b)(1)(D)).

[38] As previously noted, school food authorities may continue providing free and reduced-price meals to children enrolled in accredited academic summer school programs through the NSLP and SBP. Under the National School Lunch Act, in general, children are eligible for free meals if their families have incomes at or below 130 percent of the federal poverty guidelines and reduced-price meals if their families have incomes between 130 and 185 percent of the federal poverty guidelines.

[39] Forty-one states responded to both our questions about school food authority participation in the Seamless Summer Option and SFSP, of which 34 reported greater school food authority participation in the SFSP, 3 reported greater school food authority participation in the Seamless Summer Option, and 4 reported equal school food authority participation in the SFSP and the Seamless Summer Option. According to FNS officials, the information it collects does not separate the number of school food authorities from the number of school sponsors participating in the SFSP. Additionally, the information FNS collects on the number of school food authorities participating in the NSLP and SBP does not separate out those school food authorities specifically participating in the Seamless Summer Option.

[40] Meals served under the Seamless Summer Option are reimbursed at the free meal rates for the NSLP and SBP. Supper meals are reimbursed at the NSLP's free lunch rate. School food authorities that serve meals as sponsors under the SFSP generally receive slightly higher meal reimbursement rates than those operating the Seamless Summer Option. For example, school food authorities participating in the SFSP in the 48 contiguous states and D.C. were typically reimbursed $3.69 per lunch served in summer 2016, and in the Seamless Summer Option, up to $3.30 per lunch served before July and up to $3.39 per lunch served beginning in July.

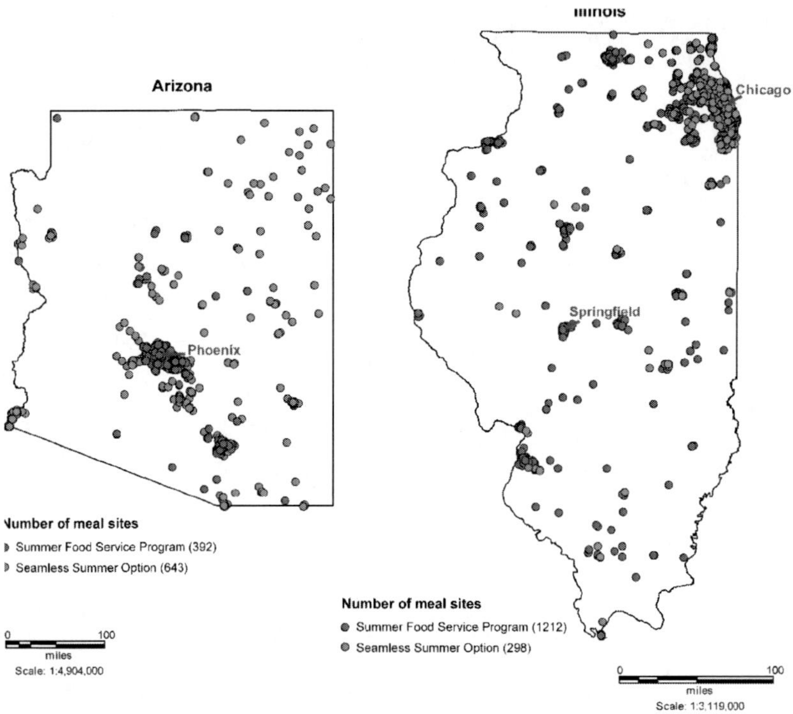

Source: GAO analysis of site level data provided by Arizona and Illinois state agency officials. MapInfo (map). | GAO-18-369.

Figure 3. Seamless Summer Option and Summer Food Service Program (SFSP) Meal Sites in Arizona (June 2016) and in Illinois (July 2016).

In summer 2016, the Seamless Summer Option added to the geographic availability of summer meal sites in two of the three states we visited as part of our review. School food authorities provided summer meals through the Seamless Summer Option in Arizona and Illinois, but not in Massachusetts, based on our analysis of data provided by these states. In Arizona and Illinois, school food authorities participating in the Seamless Summer Option added 643 and 298 summer meal sites, respectively, in the month with the largest number of SFSP meals served in each state (see Figure 3).[41] In addition, some of the Seamless Summer

---

[41] The months with the largest number of SFSP meals served are June in Arizona and July in Illinois, according to Arizona and Illinois state officials. As noted earlier, state agency officials and sponsors we spoke with in Arizona explained that schools typically end the

Option sites in these two states provided meals to children in areas where there were no SFSP sites. For example, Seamless Summer Option sites provided meals in areas near the northeastern and southwestern corners of Arizona that lacked nearby SFSP sites.

In addition to the SFSP and the Seamless Summer Option, the Summer Electronic Benefit Transfer for Children (Summer EBT) demonstration provided nutrition assistance benefits to 209,000 low-income children in summer 2016 in select areas across 6 states and 2 Indian Tribal Organizations, according to FNS officials.[42] Since the summer of 2011, Summer EBT benefits have been provided to eligible households on an electronic benefits transfer card, which households use to purchase eligible foods at authorized retailers.[43] Specifically, the demonstration has provided monthly benefits of $30 or $60 per eligible child to households with children in areas with a perceived high level of need, based on the demonstration grantees' assessments of the percentage of children eligible for free or reduced-price school meals and the availability of the SFSP.[44]

---

academic year in May, with some schools returning to session in July, and therefore, June is the busiest month for SFSP in Arizona. On the other hand, officials in Illinois explained that the SFSP usually serves the most meals in July because the academic year in that state typically ends in late June.

[42] According to FNS officials, eight grantees participated in the Summer EBT demonstrations in 2016: Cherokee Nation, Chickasaw Nation, Connecticut, Delaware, Michigan, Missouri, Nevada, and Oregon.

[43] Summer EBT benefits have been provided to households through the existing electronic benefits transfer (EBT) systems for either the Supplemental Nutrition Assistance Program (SNAP) or the Special Supplemental Nutrition Program for Women, Infants, and Children (WIC). The demonstration benefits followed the general program rules of either SNAP or WIC, depending upon the model selected by each state or Indian Tribal Organization. In the sites using the SNAP EBT systems to deliver Summer EBT benefits, participants could redeem benefits for SNAP-eligible foods at any SNAP-authorized retailer in the nation; whereas, in the sites using the WIC EBT system to deliver these benefits, participants could redeem benefits only for a limited set of foods and only at WIC-authorized retailers.

[44] As described earlier in this chapter, the Agriculture, Rural Development, Food and Drug Administration, and Related Agencies Appropriations Act, 2010, appropriated funds for USDA to develop and test methods of providing access to food for low-income children in urban and rural areas during the summer months when schools are not in regular session. Pub. L. No. 111-80, § 749(g), 123 Stat. 2090, 2132-33. Subsequent appropriations acts continued to fund these demonstrations, most recently the Consolidated Appropriations Act, 2018, Pub. L. No. 115-141, div. A, tit. IV, 132 Stat. 348. FNS developed a multi-phased demonstration approach to test different strategies to improve program participation—both enhancements to the existing SFSP and new ways of providing nutrition assistance to children in the summer. The Summer EBT was one of the new approaches tested. According to FNS officials, the design of the Summer EBT demonstrations, including

Consistent with this, three of the states that participated in Summer EBT in 2016 reported through our survey that these benefits helped children who were unable to access summer meals through the SFSP or the Seamless Summer Option. Further, according to an FNS-funded evaluation, Summer EBT improved food security among low-income children who participated in the demonstration. Specifically, the evaluation found the receipt of these benefits reduced the number of children in the demonstration experiencing very low food security between 2011 and 2013 by one-third.[45]

Some low-income children also receive nutrition assistance in the summer through federal programs that operate year-round. According to FNS data, in June 2016, 5.8 million infants and children participated in the Special Supplemental Nutrition Program for Women, Infants, and Children (WIC) and 3 million children participated in the Child and Adult Care Food Program (CACFP).[46] In addition, an average of 19.2 million children participated each month in the Supplemental Nutrition Assistance Program (SNAP) in fiscal year 2016, according to FNS data.[47] These benefits are provided year-round, including when school is in session and children may

---

benefit amounts and the number of participating grantees and children, was determined by a number of factors, including research and evaluation needs, the capacity of the grantees that operate the demonstrations, and available funding. In summer 2017, seven states and two Indian Tribal Organizations participated in the Summer EBT demonstration, according to FNS officials.

[45] Abt Associates, Inc., Mathematica Policy Research, and Maximus, Summer Electronic Benefit Transfer for Children *(SEBTC) Demonstration: Summary Report*. (May 2016). The evaluation found that 9.1 percent of the eligible households that did not receive Summer EBT benefits experienced very low food security for children from 2011 through 2013 compared to 6.1 and 6.7 percent of the eligible households that received a $60 or $30 per child per month Summer EBT benefit, respectively, over the same time period. Very low food security was measured using a survey module developed by USDA to assess and monitor food security in large-scale population studies and was defined as a circumstance when "the food intake of household members is reduced and their normal eating patterns are disrupted because the household lacks money and other resources for food." Since the demonstration was limited to select locations and households, the findings from the evaluation are not generalizable nationwide.

[46] WIC provides low-income pregnant, breastfeeding, and postpartum women, as well as infants and children up to age 5, who are determined to be at nutritional risk with supplemental foods, nutrition education, and health care referrals. The CACFP provides aid to child and adult care institutions and family or group day care homes for the provision of nutritious foods that contribute to the wellness, healthy growth, and development of young children, and the health and wellness of older adults and chronically impaired disabled persons.

[47] SNAP provides monthly benefits to low-income households which may be used to purchase food at authorized retail stores.

also be eligible to receive school meals. In our previous work on federal domestic food assistance programs, we reported that no one program alone is intended to meet a household's full nutritional needs.[48] At that time, several officials and providers told us that the variety of food assistance programs offers eligible individuals and households different types of assistance and can help households fill the gaps and address the specific needs of individual members. For example, a mother with two children may rely on SNAP for her household's basic groceries, the NSLP to feed a school-age child during the school year, and WIC to obtain supplemental foods for herself and an infant.

NONFEDERAL PROGRAMS ALSO HELP FEED LOW-INCOME CHILDREN IN THE SUMMER, BUT STATES AND LOCAL ORGANIZATIONS REPORTED THAT THESE HAVE LIMITED REACH

Some low-income children also receive summer meals through nonfederal programs, according to our state survey and interviews with organizations involved in summer meals. Twenty-seven states reported in our survey that they were aware of other state- or non-state-funded programs that provided children of low-income households with meals in their states during the summer months.[49]

According to our analysis of state survey responses, local faith-based organizations and foodbanks were the most common types of entities operating these types of programs.

---

[48] GAO, *Domestic Food Assistance: Complex System Benefits Millions, but Additional Efforts Could Address Potential Inefficiency and Overlap among Smaller Programs*, GAO-10-346 (Washington, D.C.: April 2010); and *Domestic Food Assistance: Multiple Programs Benefit Millions of Americans, but Additional Action Is Needed to Address Potential Overlap and Inefficiencies*, GAO-15-606T (Washington, D.C.: May 2015).

[49] Our survey question asked states to include programs that provide food as a secondary benefit, programs where food is the primary purpose of the program, and year-long programs.

Similarly, officials from FNS and two regional organizations we interviewed said they were aware of children receiving summer meals through nonfederal programs operated by faith-based and other community organizations. In addition, SFSP site operators at 6 of the 30 meal sites we visited in the selected states told us nearby foodbanks and faith-based organizations may also be providing children with free meals to some extent. For example, one of the meal sites we visited was operated by a foodbank that, in addition to the SFSP, provided food boxes to those in need and distributed food to other local community organizations to provide to persons in need of immediate assistance, including families with children.

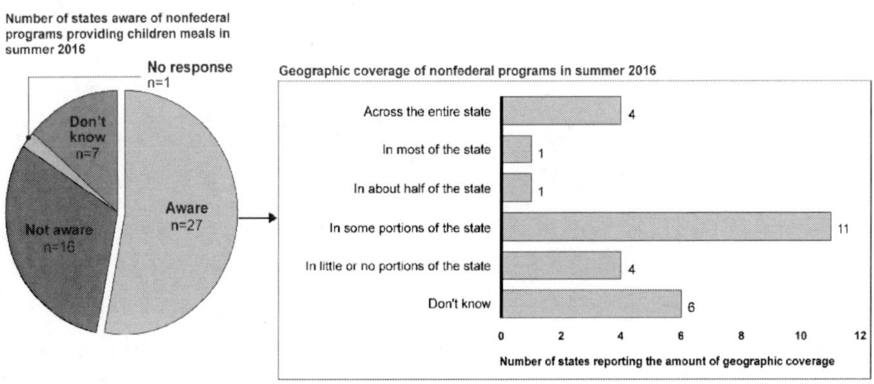

Source: GAO analysis of responses from its survey of state agencies responsible for administering the Summer Food Service Program. GAO obtained responses from 50 states and the District of Columbia. | GAO-18-369.

Figure 4. State Reported Awareness and Geographic Coverage of Nonfederal Programs Providing Meals to Children in Summer 2016.

Although FNS and the majority of states do not collect data on nonfederal programs, results from our state survey and interviews with SFSP providers and organizations involved in summer meals indicate the reach of nonfederal programs is limited.[50]

---

[50] As previously noted, throughout our report, references to "SFSP providers" include both sponsors of SFSP sites and meal site operators, if different from the sponsor.

In our survey, states reported that the geographic coverage of these nonfederal programs varied by state, with 11 states indicating that they operated in some portions of the state—the most common state response. In addition, 16 states reported that they were not aware of any nonfederal programs providing summer meals to children in their state (see Figure 4). Similarly, SFSP site operators at 24 of the 30 meal sites we visited were unaware of nonfederal programs providing meals to children in the areas in which they operated. In addition, officials from several national organizations involved in summer meals told us children have very few options for receiving summer meals beyond the federal summer meals programs. Specifically, officials from one national organization explained that food is often a significant part of the cost of a summer activity program for children and suggested that is one reason why organizations choose to participate in the SFSP.

Although the SFSP provides for federal reimbursement of eligible meals and certain administrative and operating costs, nonfederal programs that provide children with summer meals may choose not to participate in the SFSP for several reasons, according to officials we interviewed from several organizations involved in summer meals. For example, some nonfederal program providers may not participate in the SFSP because they are unaware the program exists. Additionally, some nonfederal program providers may be aware of the SFSP, but choose not to participate because they do not want to follow certain program requirements, such as the nutrition or meal pattern standards. In addition, some providers may not participate in the program because they do not think they can handle certain aspects of the administrative workload associated with the SFSP. For example, a state official we interviewed told us the administrative workload associated with the SFSP can be particularly challenging, especially for smaller sponsors. Similarly, officials from a regional organization involved in summer meals told us one of the providers they work with who operated 10 meal sites chose to leave the SFSP because the paperwork required to operate the sites was too administratively burdensome for their volunteer site operators.

STATES AND SFSP PROVIDERS FACE CHALLENGES WITH MEAL SITES, PARTICIPATION, AND PROGRAM ADMINISTRATION, AND FNS ACTIONS HAVE ADDRESSED SOME, BUT NOT ALL AREAS

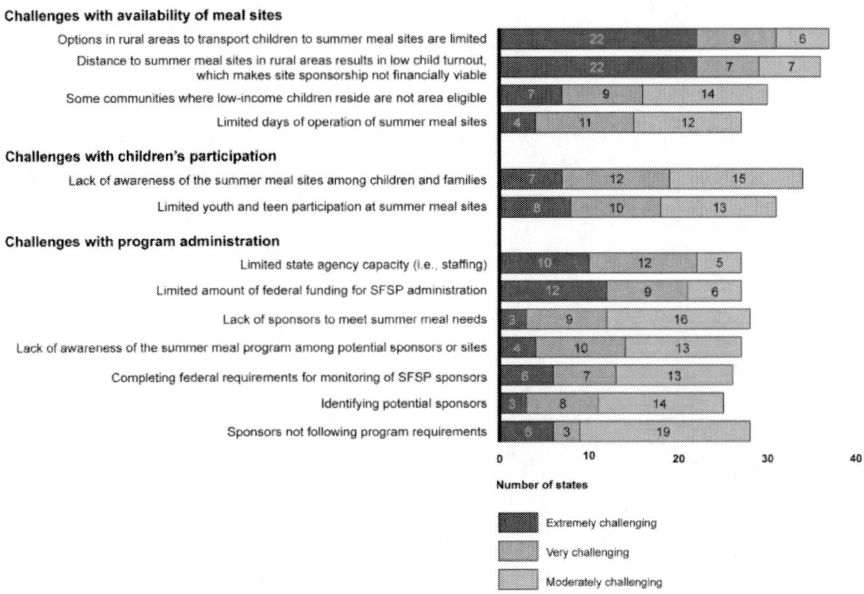

Source: GAO analysis of responses from its survey of state agencies responsible for administering the Summer Food Service Program. GAO obtained responses from 50 states and the District of Columbia. | GAO-18-369.

Note: Respondents from some states also reported these factors as slightly challenging or not at all. In addition, fewer than half of states reported other factors as moderately to extremely challenging.

Figure 5. Issues Reported as a Moderate to Extreme Challenge with the Summer Food Service Program (SFSP) by Half or More of States in GAO's Survey.

States and SFSP providers reported challenges with meal sites, participation, and administration, though federal, state, and local entities have taken steps to improve these areas. Half or more of states reported in our survey that SFSP issues related to meal site availability, such as in rural areas, increasing children's participation, and program administration were moderately to extremely challenging (see Figure 5).[51] Overall, 41 states reported facing at least one challenge with the SFSP, while 9 reported facing none.[52]

Challenges with the Availability of Meal Sites

Rural Areas

Availability of transportation, low population density, and limited meal sites pose challenges for SFSP in rural areas, according to states we surveyed, selected national organizations, and state and local officials in the three selected states we visited. More than two-thirds of states in our survey reported they faced a moderate to extreme challenge with limited options in rural areas to transport children to summer meal sites (37), as well as with the distance to summer meal sites in rural areas resulting in low child turnout that affects the financial viability of site sponsorship (36). As officials from one national organization explained, it may not be cost-effective for sponsors to operate in remote or rural areas if there are not enough meal sites or children participating in the program. Similarly, a sponsor in one of the selected states indicated that there are large parts of the state where the distances between meal sites are substantial, and travel between them takes several hours. An official from one of the selected states said transportation challenges can lead to underserved rural areas, including Indian reservations. Of the three states we reviewed, each had rural areas with few or no federally funded meal sites in summer 2016. However, a majority of the children in some of those areas were eligible for free or reduced price school meals, according to Census data provided by FNS, and would therefore be "area eligible" for the purposes of SFSP.[53]

---

[51] Some states also reported these factors as slightly challenging. In addition, fewer than half of states reported other factors as moderately to extremely challenging. See appendix II for more information on our survey results.

[52] One state in our survey did not respond to our question on experiencing challenges with administering the SFSP.

[53] See appendix III for additional information, including a map of each of the three selected states we visited.

For example, as shown in figure 6, “area eligible” locations in rural western parts of Arizona did not have any SFSP or Seamless Summer Option meals sites in June 2016, the month with the greatest number of summer meals served in that state.[54]

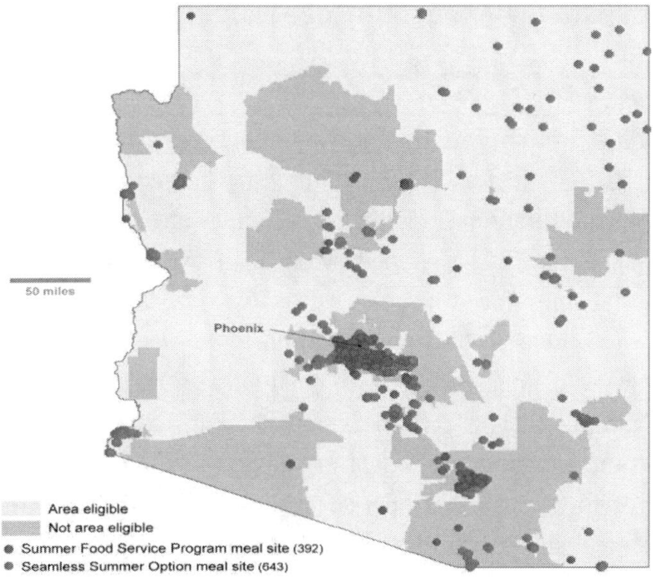

Source: GAO map based on fiscal year 2016 meal site data from Arizona on the Summer Food Service Program (SFSP) and the National School Lunch Program’s Seamless Summer Option meal sites for the month with the greatest number of meals served in Arizona (June) and area eligibility data from the Census Bureau’s American Community Survey provided by Food and Nutrition Service for fiscal year 2016. MapInfo (map). | GAO-18-369.

Note: This figure shows area eligibility as determined by the Food and Nutrition Service’s Capacity Builder mapping tool, which is based on the U.S. Census Bureau’s American Community Survey estimates of children eligible for free and reduced-price meals by Census block group and tract. However, states and sponsors may use other data to determine whether sites are “area eligible.” In addition, certain types of sites may participate in the SFSP and Seamless Summer Option even if they are not area eligible.

Figure 6. Area Eligibility and Summer Meal Sites in Arizona, June 2016.

[54] One state official in Illinois told us there are 13 counties in southern Illinois without sponsors or meal sites.

States and SFSP providers have responded to challenges with meal sites in rural areas by using other meal delivery approaches—efforts that FNS has supported through information sharing and grants.[55] For example, according to one national organization involved in summer meals, some SFSP providers offer vans or buses to transport children to meal sites or partner with local bus authorities to give children free rides to meal sites.[56] Instead of transporting children to sites, other sponsors transport meals to children through mobile meal delivery, an alternative summer meal model used in 48 states according to our survey. In this model, sponsors deliver meals by bus, using a route with state-approved stops in a community, and children consume the meal at the stop under a supervised setting. According to FNS officials and representatives from national organizations, this approach can be particularly helpful for providing summer meals to children in rural areas. State officials in two selected states told us they use mobile meal delivery to help fill gaps in meal service and help children overcome the lack of transportation or resources in their community.[57] To serve children in very remote areas with limited resources, a sponsor in one of the selected states reported piloting a model involving delivering frozen meals every other week to such areas and supplying equipment, such as freezers and microwaves, to support meal service. To help sponsors address challenges related to meal sites in rural areas, FNS has shared information on alternative delivery models through its SFSP toolkit and webinars and has also provided related grant funding. For example, in summer 2011 and 2012, FNS funded the Meal Delivery demonstration project to provide meals to children in rural areas where low population density, long distances, and transportation issues made it difficult for children to get to SFSP sites, making site and sponsor

---

[55] Throughout our report, references to "SFSP providers" include both sponsors of SFSP sites and meal site operators, if different from the sponsor.

[56] Federal reimbursement is available for SFSP operating costs, which may include the cost of transporting children in rural areas to feeding sites in rural areas. 7 C.F.R. § 225.2.

[57] FNS officials explained it can be challenging to keep children at the mobile route's stop long enough to consume the meal and qualify for federal reimbursement. To help keep children engaged during the stop and ensure they consume the meal on site, SFSP providers offer physical activities and prizes, according to one sponsor we interviewed. Another sponsor in one selected state said their library mobile reading model combines the library's mobile book service with bringing meals to children.

operation financially unsustainable.[58] The demonstration project funded meals to children in rural areas of Delaware, Massachusetts, and New York, providing food delivery to homes or drop-off sites near homes of eligible children.[59]

Area Eligibility

More than half the states (30) in our survey reported they faced a moderate to extreme challenge reaching low-income children in communities that are not area eligible. Areas in which fewer than 50 percent of children qualify for free or reduced-price meals during the school year are not eligible to have open summer meal sites at which all children who come to the site can receive a free meal. As a result, some children who are eligible for free and reduced-price meals during the school year do not have open summer meal sites located in close proximity to their residences, according to several national organization officials and SFSP providers. Eligible children in these areas may instead be limited to other types of SFSP sites, such as closed enrolled summer meal sites, or nonfederal programs providing meals, if available.[60] For example, in one of

---

[58] These projects were carried out under USDA's demonstration authority discussed earlier, which was first established by the Agriculture, Rural Development, Food and Drug Administration, and Related Agencies Appropriations Act, 2010. The act appropriated $85 million to develop and test methods of providing access to food for low-income children in urban and rural areas during the summer months when schools are not in regular session, to reduce or eliminate the food insecurity and hunger of low-income children and improve their nutritional status. Subsequent appropriations acts have continued to provide funding for demonstrations. FNS developed a multi-phased demonstration approach to test different strategies to improve program participation—both enhancements to the existing SFSP, known as eSFSP demonstrations, and new ways of providing nutrition assistance to low-income children in the summer, such as the Summer EBT.

[59] States applying for the meal delivery project were required to select sites in rural areas. According to a 2013 FNS report evaluating the eSFSP demonstrations, FNS reported that enhancements to the SFSP appeared to reach the targeted low-income children, although the reach remained limited. Furthermore, the report found that the demonstrations' impact on food security remained unclear. *Report on the Summer Food for Children Demonstration Projects for Fiscal Year 2013, U.S. Department of Agriculture Food and Nutrition Service, A Report to Congress*, December 2013.

[60] Closed enrolled sites limit participation to children enrolled in a program. All enrolled children receive free meals as long as at least 50 percent of the children enrolled meet the income eligibility standards. Eligibility for closed enrolled sites is determined through applications completed by household members on behalf of the child enrolled, or other sources of information that can be used to determine site eligibility, such as school or census data.

the selected states, a sponsor of SFSP sites funded meals without federal support at one site that they operated as an open site in order to serve low-income children residing in low-income housing. These children did not otherwise have access to a federally funded summer meals site, according to these officials, because the broader area was part of a school district that had a greater than 50 percent proportion of children from higher-income families.

Recognizing that some children may reside in an area that is not area eligible but is immediately adjacent to such an area, FNS has allowed additional flexibility in establishing area eligibility for open meal sites. Specifically, in 2014 and 2016 policy memos, FNS expanded the ways in which states and sponsors can use Census data to establish area eligibility. For example, FNS has allowed states and sponsors to average Census data across adjacent geographic areas to determine area eligibility.[61] FNS noted that these additional flexibilities help ensure meal sites can be located in more areas in which poor economic conditions exist.

Limited Days of Operation

Nearly all states (50) reported in our survey that the availability of meal sites throughout the summer months was a factor critical to the success of the SFSP, yet more than half the states (27) also reported they faced a moderate to extreme challenge with limited meal site days of operation. Nineteen of the 40 states that provided information about site days of operation reported 1 day as the shortest length of operation for SFSP sites in their state in fiscal year 2016.[62] Limited meal site days of

---

According to officials from one national organization involved in summer meals, there are relatively few closed enrolled sites that serve income-eligible children.

[61] SP 08-2017, CACFP 04-2017, SFSP 03-2017: *Area Eligibility in Child Nutrition Programs*, December 1, 2016. SP 49-2014, CACFP 13-2014, SFSP 19-2014: *Area Eligibility Using Census Data,* May 28, 2014. According to FNS, up to three adjacent census block groups may be averaged, using a weighted average, to determine eligibility. Meal sites are considered area eligible if the percentage of children eligible for free or reduced-price meals in the "referent" census block group and up to two additional adjacent census block groups, when averaged, is 50 percent or more, provided that at least 40 percent of children in each of the census block groups are eligible for free or reduced-price meals.

[62] Nineteen states reflect the highest frequency of responses provided by states responding to this survey question. In addition, 11 states reported the shortest operation among their SFSP sites was 5 days. The remaining 10 states reported the shortest number of days of operation

operation was a significant challenge in one of the three selected states we visited, as almost one-quarter of sites operated for only 1 to 2 weeks across a 2-month period in summer 2016, and an additional half of sites operated for 3 to 4 weeks across that same period, according to our analysis of state data.[63] In contrast, in the other two selected states, the majority of sites (64 and 76 percent, respectively) operated for 5 or more weeks during a 2-month period. SFSP sites may have limited days of operation for various reasons, such as constraints with program administration and costs, according to interviews with a national organization official and a sponsor in one of the selected states.

Some SFSP providers and national organizations involved in summer meals have responded to these challenges by working to extend the days of operation of meal sites—efforts that FNS has supported through related grant funding. Officials from one meal site located at a school in one of the selected states told us that 2017 was the first year the site stayed open an additional 4 weeks after summer school classes ended in an effort to expand participation, an extension made possible through support from an experienced sponsor. In addition, officials from a national organization involved in sponsoring summer meals told us they encourage their local sites to operate in August—a month where there are generally fewer summer meal service offerings—to meet children's needs. At the federal level, under its demonstration authority, FNS funded the Extending Length of Operation Incentive project, a grant which provided an additional 50-cent reimbursement for all lunch meals served at sites in Arkansas in 2010 that offered meals for 40 or more days.[64]

---

in the range of 3 to 81 days. According to officials from one national organization involved in the SFSP, meal sites operating for 1 day may be onetime events. Such one-time or special events could include a summer kick-off event in the community to help promote awareness of the program.

[63] Our analysis of selected state data on meal sites was for June, July, and August 2016. In our analysis, weeks were measured as 5 days instead of 7.

[64] According to a 2013 FNS report evaluating the eSFSP demonstrations, FNS reported that enhancements to the SFSP appeared to reach the targeted low-income children, although the reach remained limited. Furthermore, the report found that the demonstrations' impact on food security remained unclear. *Report on the Summer Food for Children Demonstration Projects for Fiscal Year 2013, U.S. Department of Agriculture Food and Nutrition Service, A Report to Congress* (December 2013).

Challenges with Children's Participation

Awareness of the SFSP Program and Meal Sites

Two-thirds of states (34) reported through our survey that they also faced a moderate to extreme challenge with a lack of awareness of summer meal sites among children and families, a challenge also mentioned by SFSP providers in the selected states. Meal site operators in one selected state noted that making families aware that all children may receive a meal for free at open sites can be a challenge. For example, one sponsor operating a meal site in a school said the perception among some is that the meal program is only for children attending summer school, and not for others in the community. Although that site had outside banners and advertising to help address that misperception, another SFSP provider explained that having sufficient funds to market the SFSP and increase awareness among families is also a challenge.[65]

To address these challenges, state agencies, some SFSP providers, and FNS have taken steps to help promote awareness of the SFSP. For example, nearly all states (47) reported in our survey that they have increased their outreach efforts for the SFSP in the last 5 years. More than half of states (36) also reported increases in overall SFSP participation during that time, which they believe were related to their outreach efforts. The majority of states in our survey reported conducting outreach on the SFSP to groups including children, parents and guardians, and schools, among others, using methods such as flyers, email, newspapers, and social media (see Figure 7).[66] Further, state agency officials and sponsors in the selected states reported that they have developed partnerships with state and local advocacy groups and community leaders, among others, to promote the SFSP. For example, one state agency official said they partner with local advocacy organizations to field calls from parents seeking information about summer meal sites through their hunger hotline. FNS

---

[65] Federal reimbursement also includes funds for some administrative costs, such as for planning, organizing, and managing a food service under the program.

[66] States in our survey also reported conducting outreach on the SFSP to other groups, including potential sponsor organizations and sites, and governments.

has promoted the use of such partnerships, as well as traditional and social media, to raise awareness of the SFSP. In addition, FNS developed the Summer Meals Site Finder, an online mapping tool that provides information on summer meal sites nationwide.[67]

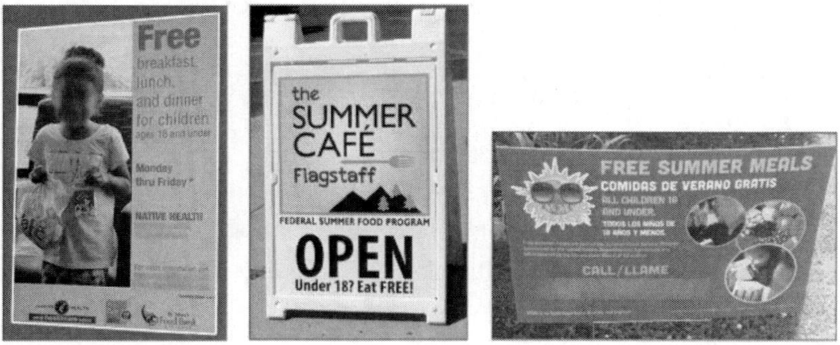
Free
breakfast,
lunch,
and dinner
for children
Monday
thru Friday*
the
SUMMER
CAFÉ
Flagstaff
FEDERAL SUMMER FOOD PROGRAM
OPEN
Under 18? Eat FREE!
FREE SUMMER MEALS
COMIDAS DE VERANO GRATIS
CALL/LLAME

Poster advertising free summer meals at health clinic meal site.

A-frame advertising of SFSP open meal site.

Lawn sign advertising free summer meals in English and Spanish.

Source: GAO. | GAO-18-369.

Figure 7. Examples of Marketing and Advertising Methods Used at Summer Food Service Program (SFSP) Meal Sites in Selected States.

Youth and Teen Participation

Attracting children of all ages to SFSP meal sites can also be a challenge, according to states and SFSP providers. More than half of the states (31) reported in our survey that they faced a moderate to extreme challenge with limited youth and teen participation at summer meal sites, and an official from a national organization involved in the SFSP explained that it is difficult to attract children to a meal site when the site is focused solely on food. Similarly, 46 states in our survey reported that providing age-appropriate programming and enrichment activities for children at summer meal sites is a factor critical to the success of the SFSP. However, some meal sites may lack the resources to add activities,

[67] The Summer Meals Site Finder is a web-based application developed by FNS to help children, parents, and others quickly and easily find summer meal sites near them. The mapping tool allows users to enter an address, city, state, or zip code to find up to 50 nearby locations, along with their addresses, hours of operation, contact information, and directions. According to FNS officials, information in the Summer Meals Site Finder is voluntarily submitted to FNS by states.

according to some SFSP providers in the selected states as well as FNS and national organization officials. Attracting teens can be particularly challenging, in part because of meal service time periods, a lack of age-appropriate activities, and stigma, according to national organizations and providers we interviewed. For example, early morning meal sites generally attract younger kids as teens may be apt to sleep later in the summer, and teens may also perceive a stigma in participating in a free meal program and may face peer pressure not to eat. In addition, meal offerings at SFSP sites may also present challenges to teen participation. Specifically, because FNS bases minimum portion size requirements for meals on the needs of younger children, meals are not always adequate to meet the nutritional needs of teens, according to one sponsor we interviewed.[68] Across the 30 meal sites in the 3 states we visited in summer 2016, we observed variety in the meals served during different meal services. (see Figure 8.)

Spotlight on Cops N Kids Program in Massachusetts

The Cops N Kids Program is a year-round effort by a local police department in Massachusetts to reduce juvenile delinquencies and to build stronger relationships with local youths. Also serving as a Summer Food Service Program (SFSP) site, Cops N Kids partnered with Project Bread, a nonprofit organization, to provide breakfast and lunch to children participating in the program. Programming at the site includes basketball, nutrition programs, and community gardening, among others. According to the sponsor of this program, their site serves between 130 and 140 meals a day.

Source: Information gathered during visit with Cops N Kids meal site in Massachusetts. | GAO-18-369.

---

[68] SFSP regulations allow sponsors to serve children age 12 and older larger portions based on the greater food needs of older children. 7 C.F.R. § 225.16(d). According to FNS guidance, sponsors may serve teenagers the adult-size portions found in the CACFP regulations, 7 C.F.R. § 226.20(c). The guidance also notes that extra food may always be served to improve the nutrition of participating children; however, meals containing additional foods or larger portion sizes than the minimum required serving size receive the same reimbursement rate as regular SFSP meals.

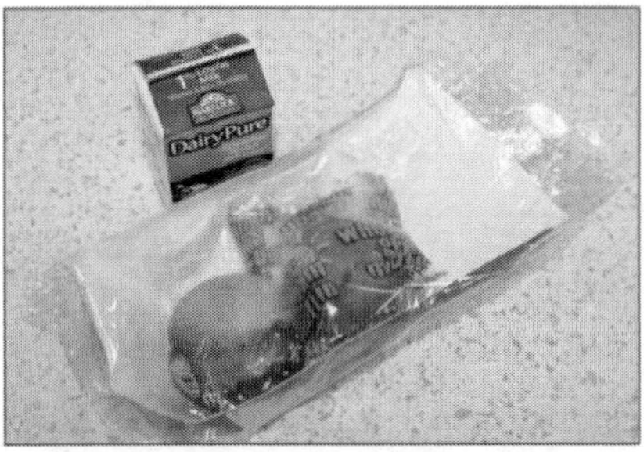

Breakfast offering of nectarine, muffin, and milk.

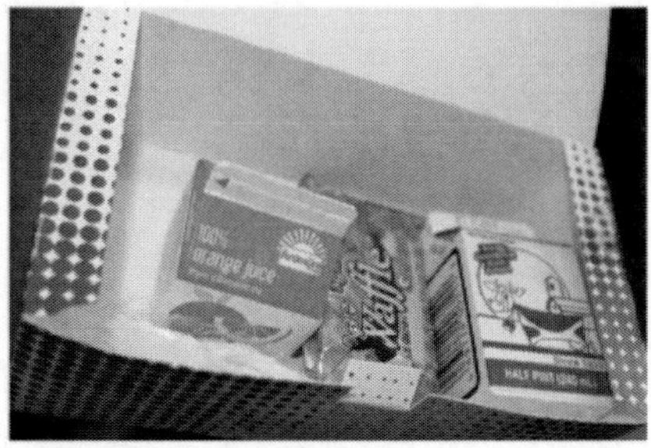

Breakfast offering of juice, waffle, and milk.

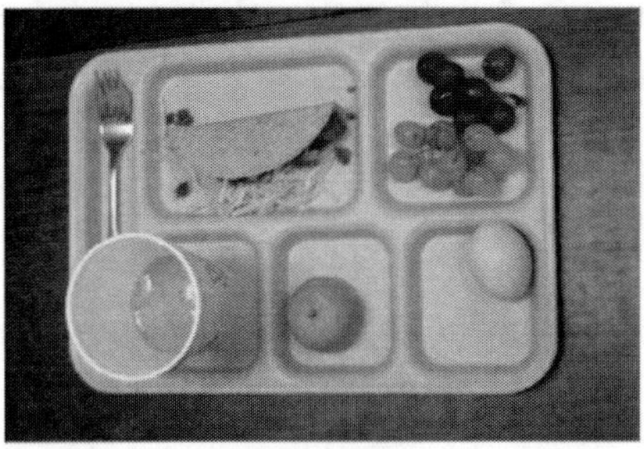

Lunch offering of taco, grapes, hard-boiled egg, clementine, and chocolate milk.

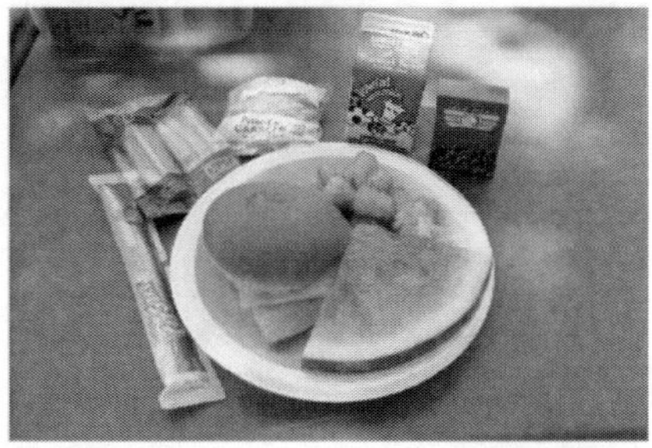

Lunch offering of ham and cheese sandwich, tater tots, watermelon, raisins, milk, carrots, and fruit popsicle.

Source: GAO. | GAO-18-369.

Figure 8. Examples of Summer Food Service Program (SFSP) Meals Served in Selected States.

States and SFSP providers have collaborated with others and sought specific types of sites to help provide enrichment activities and attract certain age groups—efforts that FNS has supported through information sharing and related grant funding. Sponsors in the selected states said they have focused on partnerships with groups such as those focused on youth development, churches, libraries, and police or fire departments, to offer age-appropriate activities for children (see Figure 9). For example, programs with local police departments, such as Cops N Kids in one selected state, or libraries in two selected states, provided meal services in combination with youth development or other enrichment activities. (See sidebar for highlights on the Cops N Kids program.) One national organization official said activities at SFSP sites can help take away the stigma around the program because children are not just there for the meal. Efforts to rebrand the SFSP as a community event where entire families can participate at the meal site also can have this effect, which is why some sponsors in the selected states said they partnered with foodbanks to donate meals for adults. In addition, a sponsor in one selected state told us they adjusted their meal offerings to match the needs of children of different age groups, for example, by serving meals to younger children earlier in the day and meals to teens later in the day.[69] To support participation from children of all ages, FNS has shared information on age-appropriate activities through its SFSP toolkit and provided related grant funding. For example, in 2010, FNS funded the Activity Incentive demonstration project, in which sponsors in Mississippi were provided with mini-grants to increase enrichment and recreational activities, such as education, tutoring, sports and games, arts and other activities, to draw children to meal sites.

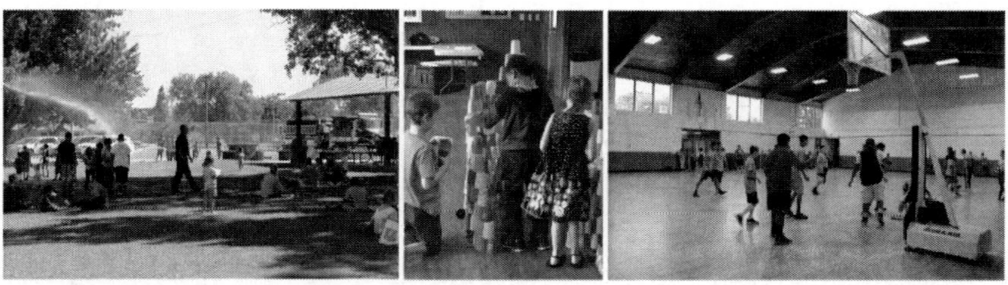

Partnership with local fire department to provide water activities for children at a Summer Food Service Program site in Arizona.

Children playing games at a Summer Food Service Program site in Illinois.

Youth and teens playing basketball at a Summer Food Service Program site in Massachusetts.

Source: GAO. | GAO-18-369.

Figure 9. Examples of Activities Offered for Children at Summer Food Service Program Meal Sites in Selected States.

Challenges with Program Administration

More than half the states reported in our survey that they faced a moderate to extreme challenge with limited state agency staffing (27), a limited amount of federal funding for SFSP administration (27), as well as

---

[69] Under SFSP requirements, sponsors generally cannot receive federal reimbursement for both lunch and supper services served on the same day. According to this sponsor, they raised other funding in order to provide teens with a supper service, in addition to the lunch service, which qualified for federal reimbursement.

ensuring sponsor participation to meet needs (28). In addition, 28 states reported in our survey that they faced a moderate to extreme challenge with sponsors not following program requirements. Limited staffing can affect a state agency's ability to conduct efforts aimed at increasing participation, identifying potential sponsors, and reviewing and monitoring sponsors, according to national organization and state officials we interviewed. For example, increases in sponsors and sites requires additional staff and time to conduct pre-approval visits, sponsor and site reviews, vendor reviews, and technical assistance visits, which directly affects the amount of funding needed to support staff salaries and travel reimbursement, according to one state in our survey. However, because the SFSP administrative funds FNS provides to states are based on the number of meals served in the previous year, increasing the number of staff to help increase SFSP participation is difficult, according to a national organization official we interviewed.[70] States reported a moderate to extreme challenge with the following issues related to ensuring sponsor participation: a lack of sponsors to meet summer meal needs, a lack of awareness of the summer meal program among potential sponsors or sites, completing federal requirements for monitoring of SFSP sponsors,[71] and identifying potential sponsors.

State agencies responsible for administering the SFSP reported relying on other resources and partners to help with program administration—strategies that FNS has supported through information sharing and its online tools. As discussed earlier, all three selected state agencies we interviewed told us they partner with advocacy groups to help expand and conduct outreach on the SFSP. Additionally, more than half the states in our survey reported several factors—which may ease the administrative

[70] Not later than February 15 of each year, each state agency must submit to FNS a program management and administration plan for that fiscal year, which includes among other things, the state's administrative budget for the year. 7 C.F.R. § 225.4 States' administrative funding amounts are calculated according to a formula that is based on the amount they received in the previous fiscal year. 7 C.F.R. § 225.5(a)(1). According to FNS officials, if states plan to expand their programs in the coming summer, it will be factored into the administrative allocation they receive.

[71] For example, states are required to conduct certain sponsor and site reviews and take corrective action when they find violations of program requirements, among other things, See 7 C.F.R. §§ 225.7(d), 225.11.

burden on states—as critical to the success of the SFSP, including partnerships with SFSP sponsors (49) and retaining sponsors and sites over multiple summers (51). To support states' use of alternative funding sources to help administer the SFSP, FNS has shared information on federal, state, and private funding and grant opportunities. FNS also developed the online Capacity Builder tool, which 35 states reported in our survey was moderately to extremely useful in identifying or confirming meal site eligibility in fiscal year 2017.[72]

States and SFSP Providers Also Reported Challenges with Meal Site Safety and Duplicative Paperwork, and FNS's Efforts to Address These Areas Are Limited

Seventeen states reported in our survey that ensuring summer meal sites are in safe locations was moderately to very challenging, a challenge that some states and SFSP providers have taken steps to help address.[73] State officials and SFSP providers in the selected states reported that when crime has occurred near a site, there are concerns about ensuring children's safety while they are consuming meals at the site, as well as the safety of site staff delivering meals. Some sponsors noted, in particular, parents' concerns for the safety of their children at meal sites in light of criminal activities in the surrounding area. To ensure children continue to have access to meals, some sponsors noted that in the event of an immediate threat at an outdoor meal site, site staff are sometimes able to bring

---

[72] The Capacity Builder tool allows users to visualize "layers" of information, such as underserved areas, and identify potential locations for new sites. Users can find their nearest potential community partners such as multi-family housing units, libraries, faith-based institutions, military bases, and schools.

[73] As noted earlier in our report, half or more of states in our survey reported facing a moderate to extreme challenge with several SFSP issues. In addition, fewer than half of states reported other factors as moderately to extremely challenging. In addition to the 17 states that reported on the issue of safe locations as moderately to very challenging, 14 states reported this issue as slightly challenging, 7 states reported this as not at all challenging, 3 states reported they did not know, and 10 states reported no response. In our survey, we did not define "safe locations." See appendix II for more information on our survey results and on the full list of challenges states reported.

children to a nearby indoor space instead. States and SFSP provider officials in two selected states told us they have also used other strategies, including partnerships with local law enforcement agencies, to help address safety concerns during the meal service and ensure children have access to meals. For example, national organizations involved in summer meals and sponsor officials in the selected states said they encourage partnerships with local police departments to use police escorts at meal sites or to follow mobile meal routes in situations where safety at the meal site is a concern. When violence or crime has occurred near a site, some states and SFSP sponsors have also sought flexibility from FNS with respect to the federal requirement that children consume summer meals on site,[74] according to state and local officials.

FNS has used its available authorities to grant some states and sponsors flexibility with respect to the requirement that children consume summer meals on site, such as when safety at the site is a concern; however, FNS has not clearly communicated to all states and sponsors the circumstances it considers when deciding whether to grant this flexibility.[75] According to our review of letters FNS sent to multiple states approving their requests for this type of flexibility, the agency identified a consistent set of circumstances that needed to be met for it to grant this flexibility.[76] These circumstances were described in the letters the agency sent to states and generally included verification that violent crime activities occurred within both a 6-block radius of the meal site and 72 hours prior to the meal service.[77] FNS's letters to states indicate that when documentation was provided to the agency showing that these circumstances existed at a summer meals site on a particular day or days, meals consumed by

---

[74] 7 C.F.R. § 225.6(e)(15).

[75] For example, FNS has granted some states and sponsors flexibility from this requirement in situations of crime or violence under its waiver and demonstration authorities. See 42 U.S.C. § 1760(l) and the Agriculture, Rural Development, Food and Drug Administration, and Related Agencies Appropriations Act, 2010, Pub. L. No. 111-80, § 749(g), 123 Stat. 2090, 2132-33, most recently funded by the Consolidated Appropriations Act, 2018, Pub. L. No. 115-141, div. A, tit. IV, 132 Stat. 348.

[76] These approvals of states' requests for flexibility were made under FNS's demonstration authority.

[77] Violent crime activities were defined in FNS's letters to states as murder, attempted murder, aggravated assault, and armed robbery.

children off site on those days were eligible for federal reimbursement.[78] Although FNS has issued guidance on the general processes for requesting flexibility from program requirements under its waiver and demonstration authorities, these guidance documents do not detail the specific circumstances that the agency considers when deciding whether to grant flexibility from the on-site requirement due to safety concerns.[79] FNS has communicated this information only in its responses to specific state and sponsor requests, and it has not communicated these circumstances more broadly to all states and sponsors. FNS officials explained that they review state and sponsor requests for flexibility due to safety concerns on a case-by-case basis. However, they also acknowledged that the set of circumstances used for approval of state and sponsor requests for flexibility, which we identified in their letters to states, has been used repeatedly.

Further, states and sponsors reported challenges obtaining the specific data needed for approval of a site for this type of flexibility, hampering some providers' efforts to ensure safe delivery of meals. For example, state agency and sponsor officials in one selected state said obtaining the crime data needed to qualify for the flexibility can be an administrative burden on sponsors, and these data are not consistently available in a timely manner. According to state agency and sponsor officials in one of the selected states, daily crime statistics are not available in all areas, and while a sponsor can sometimes access current data on crime in a city, the most

---

[78] FNS did not grant sites continued flexibility over multiple days or for the remainder of that site's operations over the summer unless the site provided such documentation for each day they requested the flexibility.

[79] For example, in its policy memo SP 14-2017, SFSP 07-2017, Demonstration Project for Non-Congregate Feeding for Outdoor Summer Meal Sites Experiencing Excessive Heat with Q&As (Jan. 2017), FNS stated that it may extend this heat-related demonstration project to other situations where exceptional circumstances make congregate meals at approved sites not viable or unsafe. The guidance further stated that such "exceptional circumstance" requests would be considered on a case-by-case basis, and that requests should clearly describe the problem, justify the need for the exception, and describe how the sponsors' operations will change and how eliminating the congregate meal requirement will address the problem. In addition, FNS also issued SP 27-2017, CACFP 12-2017, SFSP 08-2017, Child Nutrition Program Waiver Request Guidance and Protocol (Apr. 2017), which provides an overview of the statutory waiver authority, the waiver request and review process, and data reporting requirements.

recent available data on crime in suburban areas are sometimes one year old. FNS is aware of state and local challenges obtaining the necessary crime data, according to our discussions with FNS officials. FNS officials acknowledged that while they have granted some state and sponsor requests to allow children to consume meals off site in certain areas where violence or crime has occurred, some sponsors were unable to implement the flexibility because they could not obtain the necessary crime data.[80]

To help achieve agency objectives and address related risks, the *Standards for Internal Control in the Federal Government* state that agencies should communicate key information to their internal and external stakeholders.[81] Although FNS officials told us they do not have one set of circumstances under which they approve these requests, our review found only one set of circumstances under which this type of flexibility has been approved. However, FNS has not broadly communicated the circumstances it considers in deciding whether to approve requests for flexibility with respect to the requirement that children consume summer meals on site in areas with violence or crime. Unless FNS shares this information with all states and sponsors, states and sponsors will likely continue to be challenged to use this flexibility, hindering its usefulness in ensuring safe summer meal delivery to children.

In addition, FNS has issued reports to Congress evaluating some of its demonstration projects, as required under its statutory authorities, but the agency has not issued any such reports to Congress specifically on the use of flexibilities with respect to the on-site requirement in areas where safety is a concern. As previously discussed, the agency is required to annually submit certain reports to Congress regarding the use of waivers and evaluations of projects carried out under its demonstration authority.[82]

---

[80] According to the letters we reviewed approving flexibility under FNS's demonstration authority, FNS has allowed states and sponsors to use the flexibility and retroactively provide the documentation that a crime occurred within 72 hours and within 6 blocks of the meal site on that day. However, if the documentation is not available or not sufficient, the sponsor risks not being reimbursed for meals that were consumed off site that day.

[81] GAO-14-704G.

[82] Specifically, the Secretary of Agriculture is required to annually submit to the Committee on Education and Labor in the House of Representatives and the Committee on Agriculture, Nutrition, and Forestry of the Senate a report that summarizes the use of waivers and

Furthermore, *Standards for Internal Control in the Federal Government* state that management should use quality information to make informed decisions and evaluate the entity's performance in achieving key objectives and addressing risks.[83] Yet, FNS has not evaluated nor reported on the use of waivers and demonstration projects in cases where safety was a concern. Although FNS requests reports from state agencies or sponsors that have received flexibility with summer meals delivery under FNS's demonstration and waiver authorities, FNS officials told us they have not assessed whether their use of these flexibilities to address safety issues has been effective in ensuring safe meal delivery. FNS officials told us that they have not evaluated or reported on these flexibilities, in part, because they have limited information on their outcomes.[84] Without understanding the impact of its use of these flexibilities, neither FNS nor Congress knows whether these flexibilities are helping provide meals to children.

In addition to the challenges with safety at meal sites, sponsors also sometimes face administrative challenges when participating in multiple child nutrition programs that are operated by different state agencies or divisions within the same agency, according to officials from national and regional organizations and sponsors we interviewed. For example, officials from national organizations involved in summer meals told us the management of each child nutrition program and processes related to applications, funding, and oversight are fragmented in many states. For

---

describes whether they resulted in improved services to children, the impact of the waivers on providing nutritional meals to participants, and how the waivers reduced the quantity of paperwork necessary to administer the program. 42 U.S.C. § 1760(l). In addition, the Secretary is required to provide for an independent evaluation of the projects carried out under its demonstration authority, and submit annual reports to the same Committees on the status of each demonstration project and the results of the evaluations for the previous fiscal year. Further, not later than 120 days after the completion of the last evaluation, the Secretary is required to submit a report that includes recommendations on how to improve children's access to food during the summer months when school is not in regular session. See the Agriculture, Rural Development, Food and Drug Administration, and Related Agencies Appropriations Act, 2010, Pub. L. No. 111-80, § 749(g), 123 Stat. 2090, 2132-33, most recently funded by the Consolidated Appropriations Act, 2018, Pub. L. No. 115-141, div. A, tit. IV, 132 Stat. 348.

[83] GAO-14-704G.

[84] In its letters to states approving their requests for flexibility with the requirement to consume meals on-site when safety is a concern, FNS requested states and sponsors to submit reports on the implementation and results of the flexibility. However, FNS officials told us they do not always receive this information.

example, a sponsor in one of the selected states told us aspects of the SFSP and CACFP sponsor applications are highly duplicative and estimated it took 42 hours last year to complete duplicative paperwork. Another sponsor that provides school meals during the school year told us they had to fill out 60 additional pages of paperwork to provide summer meals, which coupled with having a state contact for the SFSP that was different from the one they worked with for the NSLP, was a significant burden for them. Officials from one national organization told us a lack of interoperability of some state agencies' data systems has caused challenges and administrative burden for some sponsors.[85] For example, in some states, different agencies oversee child nutrition programs, yet are unable to share data on sponsor approval, and therefore, sponsors are required to submit similar information to both, according to these officials. Duplicative paperwork can be particularly burdensome for some SFSP providers, as national organization officials and SFSP providers in the selected states said completing SFSP application paperwork can be especially challenging when a sponsor has staff shortages or no dedicated SFSP staff.

Some selected states have worked with SFSP sponsors to help minimize the administrative burden. For example, state agency officials from one of the selected states said they have connected less-experienced sponsors to more-experienced sponsors in the community to help them with program administration. In one case, an experienced SFSP sponsor partnered with a small sponsor new to the program to help with SFSP administration, including helping them understand program rules and

---

[85] In our previous work on other federal low-income programs, we reported that computer systems can be used as a tool to streamline program administration, and that data-sharing arrangements, where permitted by federal law, allow programs to share client information that they otherwise would each collect and verify separately, thus reducing duplicative effort, saving money, and improving integrity. GAO, *Federal Low-Income Programs: Eligibility and Benefits Differ for Selected Programs Due to Complex and Varied Rules*, GAO-17-558 (Washington, D.C.: June 29, 2017). In other prior work on human services programs' data sharing efforts, we also reported that some of the challenges to such data sharing included confusion or misperceptions around what data state and local agencies were allowed to share, as well as a tendency to be risk averse and overly cautious in these agencies' interpretation of federal privacy requirements. GAO, *Human Services: Sustained and Coordinated Efforts Could Facilitate Data Sharing While Protecting Privacy*, GAO-13-106, (Washington, D.C.: Feb. 8, 2013).

paperwork requirements. One SFSP sponsor also noted that their state agency took additional steps to ease administrative burden, such as making the forms for the CACFP more consistent with those for the SFSP and streamlining certain requirements for large and experienced sponsors, which the sponsor found helpful.

At the federal level, FNS has established program and policy simplifications to help lessen the administrative burden on sponsors participating in multiple child nutrition programs, though the persistence of these challenges indicate that information about these simplifications has not reached all relevant state agencies. While FNS officials told us that some of the duplicative requirements may be a function of differences in statute, FNS provided guidance to states in 2011 and 2014 on simplified application procedures for institutions participating in CACFP that also wish to apply for SFSP.[86] FNS noted in its guidance that in states where CACFP and SFSP are administered by different state agencies, state agencies are encouraged to work together to share information and streamline the application and agreement process as much as possible. FNS also addressed these simplifications in a state agency meeting in November 2017. Additionally, FNS provided guidance to states in 2012 on simplified application and review procedures for school food authorities participating in the NSLP that wish to also participate in the SFSP.[87] Although FNS has shared this information with states in an attempt to make them aware of streamlining options, FNS officials noted that some states may choose not to implement them.

Standards for Internal Control in the Federal Government state that management should externally communicate the necessary quality information to achieve the entity's objectives, as well as periodically evaluate the methods of communication to ensure communication is

---

[86] As discussed earlier, the CACFP provides aid to child and adult care institutions and family or group day care homes for the provision of nutritious foods that contribute to the wellness, healthy growth, and development of young children, and the health and wellness of older adults and chronically impaired disabled persons.

[87] SP-07-2013, SFSP-04-2013, *Summer Feeding Options for School Food Authorities* (November 2012).

effective and appropriate.[88] FNS's existing guidance addresses options for streamlining administrative requirements for sponsors participating in multiple child nutrition programs. However, information on program and policy simplifications available for sponsors participating in both NSLP and SFSP has not been shared with states recently, and challenges in this area persist, indicating this information has not reached all relevant state agencies. Without further efforts from FNS to disseminate information on current options for streamlining administrative requirements across child nutrition programs, overlapping and duplicative administrative requirements may limit children's access to meals by discouraging sponsor participation in child nutrition programs.

Conclusion

The purpose of the SFSP is to continue to provide children in low-income areas with nutritious meals over the summer when school is no longer in session, and to that end, the program provided 149 million SFSP meals to children in fiscal year 2016. Although meals served are one indicator of participation, FNS's current estimates of children participating in SFSP are unreliable. Without additional understanding of children's participation in the SFSP, FNS lacks information critical for informing program implementation, strategic planning, and outreach.

The majority of states nationwide and SFSP providers in the three states we visited reported experiencing a number of challenges with the SFSP, and FNS has taken important steps to address these challenges. Two key challenges identified by officials in the selected states and national organizations we interviewed are ensuring summer meal sites are in safe locations, and meeting administrative requirements when participating in multiple child nutrition programs. FNS has taken steps to address these challenges by providing flexibilities in how meals are delivered to children and streamlining options for those providers participating in more than one

[88] GAO-14-704G.

child nutrition program. However, a lack of clarity concerning the circumstances under which FNS grants flexibilities in areas of violence and crime, and a lack of information on its use of these flexibilities and their impact on program administration, hinder efforts to ensure program goals are met. Furthermore, absent a reminder to states regarding existing options for streamlining administration across multiple nutrition programs, some providers may continue to be discouraged from participating in these programs due to duplicative and burdensome administrative requirements, which may ultimately limit the provision of nutritious meals to children.

RECOMMENDATIONS FOR EXECUTIVE ACTION

We are making the following four recommendations to FNS:

The Administrator of FNS should improve its estimate of children's participation in the SFSP by focusing on addressing, at a minimum, data reliability issues caused by variations in the number of operating days of meal sites and in the months in which states see the greatest number of meals served. (Recommendation 1)

The Administrator of FNS should communicate to all SFSP stakeholders the circumstances it considers in approving requests for flexibility with respect to the requirement that children consume SFSP meals on-site in areas that have experienced crime and violence, taking into account the feasibility of accessing data needed for approval, to ensure safe delivery of meals to children. (Recommendation 2)

The Administrator of FNS should evaluate and annually report to Congress, as required by statute, on its use of waivers and demonstration projects to grant states and sponsors flexibility with respect to the requirement that children consume SFSP meals on-site in areas experiencing crime or violence, to improve its understanding of the use and impact of granting these flexibilities on meeting program goals. (Recommendation 3)

The Administrator of FNS should disseminate information about existing flexibilities available to state agencies to streamline administrative requirements for sponsors participating in the SFSP and other child nutrition programs to help lessen the administrative burden. For example, FNS could re-distribute existing guidance to state agencies that explains available flexibilities and encourage information sharing. (Recommendation 4)

AGENCY COMMENTS AND OUR EVALUATION

We provided a draft of this chapter to the Secretary of the USDA for review and comment. FNS officials provided technical comments, which we incorporated as appropriate. In addition, in oral comments, FNS officials, including the Deputy Administrator for Child Nutrition Programs, generally agreed with the recommendations in the report.

As agreed with your offices, unless you publicly announce the contents of this chapter earlier, we plan no further distribution until 30 days from the report date. At that time, we will send copies to the Secretary of the USDA and interested congressional committees.

Kathryn A. Larin, Director
Education, Workforce, and Income Security Issues

APPENDIX I: OBJECTIVES, SCOPE AND METHODOLOGY

This appendix discusses in detail our methodology for addressing three research objectives: (1) What is known about participation in the Summer Food Service Program (SFSP) and how has it changed in the last 10 years? (2) What other programs help feed low-income children over the summer? and (3) What challenges exist, if any, in providing summer meals to children, and to what extent does the U.S. Department of Agriculture's (USDA) Food and Nutrition Service (FNS) provide assistance to states and sponsors to address these challenges? In addition to the methods we discuss below, to address all three research objectives, we reviewed relevant federal laws, regulations, and guidance; interviewed FNS officials in its headquarters and seven regional offices; and interviewed a broad range of regional and nationwide organizations involved in the SFSP.[89] In addition, we coordinated with officials in USDA's Office of Inspector General on their ongoing work in this area.

Summer and School Meals Data

To address our first objective about participation in the SFSP, we analyzed FNS data on meals served for fiscal years 2007 through 2016.[90] Specifically, we analyzed the total number of meals served nationwide through the SFSP from fiscal year 2007 through fiscal year 2016.[91] Each month, states report to FNS the number of meals served by meal type (breakfast, lunch, snack, and supper) and the number of meals served by meal and sponsor type (e.g., government, nonprofit, etc.) using the FNS-418 form. To add context on these trends, we also analyzed and compared the number of SFSP lunches served in July with the number of free and reduced-price lunches served to children in March through the National School Lunch Program (NSLP), the largest child nutrition assistance

[89] We interviewed officials from the following organizations: Boys and Girls Club of America, Catholic Charities USA, National Child and Adult Care Food Program Sponsors Association, Feeding America, Feed the Children, Food Research & Action Center, Illinois Hunger Coalition, National League of Cities, National Recreation and Park Association, Share Our Strength, Texas Hunger Initiative, and Young Men's Christian Association (YMCA) of the USA.

[90] Our review focused on the 10 years from fiscal year 2007 through fiscal year 2016; however, we noted preliminary data from fiscal year 2017 to provide the most up-to-date information available at the time of this chapter.

[91] These data include meals served in the 50 states, American Samoa, the Commonwealth of North Marina Islands, the District of Columbia, Guam, Puerto Rico, the U. S. Virgin Islands, and U. S. Department of Defense's military bases. We only included data from the 50 states and the District of Columbia and for the months of May, June, July, and August in our review. As previously noted, our review focused on the 10 years from fiscal year 2007 through fiscal year 2016; however we noted preliminary data from fiscal year 2017 to provide the most up-to-date information available at the time of this chapter.

program, from fiscal year 2007 through fiscal year 2016.[92] Each month, states report to FNS the number of meals served through the NSLP using the FNS-10 form.[93] To assess the reliability of SFSP and NSLP data, we (1) performed electronic testing of relevant data elements, (2) reviewed existing information about the data and the system that produced them, and (3) interviewed agency officials knowledgeable about the data. Electronic testing included, but was not limited to, checks for missing data elements, duplicative records, and values outside a designated range or valid time period. We determined that these data were sufficiently reliable to identify the number of SFSP meals served and assess change over time.

To further examine what is known about participation in the SFSP, we also reviewed FNS's data on estimates of children's participation in the program and determined that these estimates have been calculated inconsistently and are unreliable. To assess the reliability of these data, we reviewed documentation about the estimates, interviewed FNS officials, and asked states about the estimate calculation in our survey. As described in our findings, FNS does not collect data on the number of children participating in the SFSP. Instead, FNS relies on states' estimates of children's participation, which are based on other data reported by sponsors, such as the number of meals served and meal service days in July.

To address our second objective about other programs that help feed children in the summer, we reviewed FNS's estimate of the number of meals served through the NSLP's Seamless Summer Option in fiscal year 2016. FNS does not collect data on the number of meals served through the Seamless Summer Option. Instead, FNS annually estimates the number of Seamless Summer Option meals served nationally by aggregating the

---

[92] The SFSP and NSLP data include meals served in the 50 states, American Samoa, the Commonwealth of North Marina Islands, the District of Columbia, Guam, Puerto Rico, the U. S. Virgin Islands, and U.S. Department of Defense's military bases. For this review, we focused our analysis on data from the 50 states and the District of Columbia. We used the month of July for the SFSP and the month of March for the NSLP because, according to FNS officials, the highest SFSP participation generally occurs in July and the highest NSLP participation generally occurs in March. FNS officials told us they generally compare these two months when comparing these two programs.

[93] The information reported for the NSLP includes the number paid, free, and reduced-price meals by meal type (e.g., lunches and snacks) for each month.

number of free and reduced-price breakfasts, lunches, and snacks served through the School Breakfast Program (SBP) and NSLP in July. As previously noted, states report these data monthly to FNS.[94] Although FNS does not know the actual number of meals served through the Seamless Summer Option, agency officials told us they believe the number of summer meals provided through the NSLP is small relative to the number of meals served through the Seamless Summer Option during the summer months. They noted that their use of July NSLP data to estimate the Seamless Summer Option meals likely overestimates the number of these meals for July and underestimates the number of these meals for the entire summer. To assess the reliability of the July NSLP data, we (1) performed electronic testing of relevant data elements, (2) reviewed existing information about the data and the system that produced them, and (3) interviewed agency officials knowledgeable about the data. Electronic testing included, but was not limited to, checking for missing data and data that fell outside of a reasonable range or date for the specific time period (July). We determined that these data were sufficiently reliable to describe the number of meals served.

In addition to the data FNS requires states to report, some states collect summer meals data at the meal site level and we used such data from the three selected states to address all three objectives. For objective one, to examine the number of meals served and days of operation at each summer meals site, we analyzed site-level data for 2 months from summer 2016, including the month with the largest number of SFSP meals served in each selected state: Arizona (June and July 2016), Illinois (July and August 2016), and Massachusetts (July and August 2016). Each state also provided us with data on the number and types of meals served at each SFSP site, the site location, and the duration of time each site operated over the summer. Using the data provided by the states, we calculated the average daily attendance (ADA) for each meal site based on FNS's instructions and examined the variation in ADA across sites and months. For our second objective on other programs, these selected states provided similar site

---

[94] The information reported for the NSLP and SBP includes the number paid, free, and reduced-price meals by meal type (e.g., snacks and breakfasts) for each month.

level data for the state's Seamless Summer Option sites, if applicable.[95] We assessed the reliability of these data by (1) performing electronic testing of relevant data elements, (2) reviewing existing information about the data and the system that produced them, and (3) interviewing agency officials knowledgeable about the data. We determined that the data were sufficiently reliable for the purposes of this chapter.

For both our second objective on other programs and third objective about challenges in providing summer meals to children, we also examined meal site availability in the three selected states by mapping the locations of meal sites. On the maps, we included fiscal year 2016 area eligibility data from FNS's Capacity Builder mapping tool, as provided by FNS.[96] The site area eligibility data from FNS's Capacity Builder is based on the U.S. Census Bureau's 5-Year American Community Survey (ACS) estimates of children ages 0-12 and 0-18 eligible for free and reduced-price meals by Census block group and tract.[97] According to FNS officials, FNS obtains 5-Year ACS estimates annually from the U.S. Census Bureau and updates its site area eligibility in the Capacity Builder accordingly. For fiscal year 2016, FNS used 2009- 2013 ACS data to identify and include site area eligibility in its Capacity Builder.[98]

Survey

To help inform all of our research objectives, we conducted a survey of the state agencies that oversee the SFSP in the 50 states and the District of

[95] School food authorities provided summer meals through the Seamless Summer Option in Arizona and Illinois, but not in Massachusetts, based on our analysis of data provided by these states.

[96] FNS's Capacity Builder is a mapping tool that allows users to search for summer meal sites from the previous summer by zip code, adding "layers" of information, such as area eligibility data.

[97] States are responsible for determining meal site eligibility and sponsors may demonstrate area eligibility using other forms of data, such as school data. Area eligibility determinations made using either school or census data must be re-determined periodically. USDA, Food and Nutrition Service, *Area Eligibility in Child Nutrition Programs,* Memo code SP 08-2017, CACFP 04-2017, SFSP 03-2017 (Alexandria, Virginia: December 1, 2016).

[98] According to FNS officials, the 2009-2013 ACS data estimates were the most recently available from the U.S. Census Bureau for fiscal year 2016.

Columbia. We administered our web-based survey between August and October 2017 and received 100 percent response rate. The survey included questions about participation in the SFSP, factors critical to the overall success of the SFSP, outreach efforts, federal technical assistance, barriers and challenges in providing summer meals, alternative summer feeding models, the NSLP's Seamless Summer Option and the federal Summer Electronic Benefit Transfer for Children demonstration, and nonfederal programs that provide children of low-income households with meals during the summer months. The survey also requested data on SFSP sites participating in the program in fiscal year 2016 and the method state agencies used to calculate ADA in SFSP on the FNS-418 form in fiscal year 2016.

Because this was not a sample survey, there are no sampling errors. However, the practical difficulties of conducting any survey may introduce nonsampling errors, such as variations in how respondents interpret questions and their willingness to offer accurate responses. We took steps to minimize nonsampling errors, including pretesting draft instruments and using a web-based administration system. Specifically, during survey development, we pretested draft instruments with SFSP staff from four states (Michigan, New Mexico, North Carolina, and South Dakota) in May 2017. We selected the pretest states based on information provided by officials from FNS's regional offices and national organizations involved in summer meals about state administration of summer meals programs, with the goal of selecting a group of states with varied experiences. In the pretests, we were generally interested in the clarity, precision, and objectivity of the questions, as well as the flow and layout of the survey. For example, we wanted to ensure definitions used in the surveys were clear and known to the respondents, categories provided in close-ended questions were complete and exclusive, and the ordering of survey sections and the questions within each section were appropriate. We revised the final survey based on pretest results. Another step we took to minimize nonsampling errors was using a web-based survey.

Allowing respondents to enter their responses directly into an electronic instrument created a record for each respondent in a data file and eliminated the need for and the errors associated with a manual data entry process. We did not fully validate specific information that states reported through our survey.

Site Visits

To help inform all of our objectives and gather information about the SFSP directly at the local-level, we conducted 30 site visits in three states: Arizona (12 sites), Illinois (8 sites), and Massachusetts (10 sites) between June and July 2017, and interviewed organizations involved with the SFSP in each site visit state. We used U.S. Census Bureau data to select states and local areas within those states based on a high proportion of children in poverty, a mix of urban and rural locations, as well as a mix of sponsor and site type and diverse locations. We visited a wide variety of site locations including, but not limited to, schools, parks, community recreation areas, and libraries.

At each SFSP site, we gathered information on local level factors related to SFSP participation and administration by interviewing the organization sponsoring the site, the site operators and staff, and those participating at the site using semi-structured questions. While interviewing SFSP sponsor organizations, we collected information on the sponsors' roles in the SFSP, characteristics of the sites the organizations sponsored, outreach efforts, any challenges or barriers to SFSP administration and any efforts to address such challenges, relationships with the state agencies that administer the SFSP, relationships with FNS (national and regional offices), and the availability of nonfederally funded programs that provide meals to low-income children over the summer.

During the interviews with site operators and staff, we collected information about site operation (e.g., site operating days, meals offered, etc.), any challenges to providing SFSP meals to children and any efforts to address such challenges, outreach efforts, and the proximity of the next closest meal site. The information we collected from those participating at the sites included their perspectives on the SFSP food, site food consumption habits, ease of travel to the site, and access to other SFSP sites. At each site, we made observations as to how the food was provided to the children, food consumption and waste, the approximate age range of the children being served, and availability of programs or activities (e.g., recreational sports).

Using semi-structured questions, we also interviewed the state agencies responsible for administering the SFSP in the site visit states to gather further information on how the SFSP is administered in each state, statewide participation in the program, related data collection activities, any challenges to administering the program and any efforts to address such challenges, related outreach efforts, alternative meal delivery models being employed by SFSP sponsors, FNS guidance or technical assistance, and the availability of nonfederally funded programs that provide meals to low-income children over the summer.

APPENDIX II: SELECT QUESTIONS AND RESPONSES FROM GAO'S SUMMER FOOD SERVICE PROGRAM (SFSP) SURVEY

Table 2. Survey Question 2: Does your state agency experience any challenges with administering the SFSP?

Prompt	Number of States Reporting
Yes	41
No	9
No Response	1

Source: Responses to GAO's survey of state agencies responsible for administering the Summer Food Service Program. | GAO-18-369

Table 3. Survey Question 2A: How challenging are the following factors to state administration of the SFSP?

Prompt	Extremely challenging	Very challenging	Moderately challenging	Slightly challenging	Not at all challenging	Not applicable	Don't know	No response
Limited state agency capacity (i.e., staffing)	10	12	5	11	2	1	0	10
Limited overall state budget	6	3	9	2	6	14	1	10
Limited amount of state funding for SFSP administration	3	3	2	2	4	25	2	10
Limited amount of federal funding for SFSP administration	12	9	6	3	8	2	1	10
Identifying potential sponsors	3	8	14	8	6	2	0	10
Conducting outreach to potential sponsors	4	5	15	11	5	1	0	10
Retaining sponsors and sites over multiple summers	2	4	14	14	5	2	0	10
Identification and confirmation of site area eligibility	1	2	10	16	10	2	0	10
Completing federal requirements for monitoring of SFSP sponsors	6	7	13	8	6	0	0	11
Other[a]	6	5	3	1	0	13	4	19

Source: Responses to GAO's survey of state agencies responsible for administering the Summer Food Service Program (SFSP). | GAO-18-369.

[a]For states that indicated there were other challenge(s), we provided an open-ended question that requested a description of the challenge(s) and 14 states provided descriptions of other challenges, not shown here.

Table 4. Survey Question 2B: How challenging are the following local-level factors to increasing children's participation in the SFSP?

Prompt	Extremely challenging	Very challenging	Moderately challenging	Slightly challenging	Not at all challenging	Don't know	No response
Lack of sponsors to meet summer meal needs	3	9	16	11	2	0	10
Some communities where low-income children reside are not area eligible	7	9	14	8	2	1	10
Distance to summer meal sites in rural areas results in low child turnout, which makes site sponsorship not financially viable for sponsors	22	7	7	2	1	2	10
Options in rural areas to transport children to summer meal sites are limited	22	9	6	1	1	2	10
Limited days of operation of summer meal sites	4	11	12	12	2	0	10
Ensuring sufficient staff supervision of children at summer meal sites	2	6	16	10	3	4	10
Ensuring summer meal sites are in safe locations	0	7	10	14	7	3	10
Lack of awareness of the summer meal sites among children and families	7	12	15	6	1	0	10
Lack of awareness of the summer meal program among potential sponsors or sites	4	10	13	13	0	1	10
Sponsors not following program requirements	6	3	19	11	2	0	10
Poor meal quality at summer meal sites	3	6	9	16	7	0	10
Inadequate meal reimbursement amounts	4	13	6	10	7	1	10
Limited youth and teen participation at summer meals sites	8	10	13	8	1	1	10
Difficulty ensuring meal sites are available throughout the summer due to unexpected changes in school calendars	3	3	11	11	10	2	11
Other[a]	5	2	1	0	1	16	26

Source: Responses to GAO's survey of state agencies responsible for administering the Summer Food Service Program (SFSP). | GAO-18-369.

[a]For states that indicated there were other challenge(s), we provided an open-ended question that requested a description of the challenge(s) and 8 states provided descriptions of other challenges, not shown here.

Appendix III: Area Eligibility and Summer Meal Sites in Selected States

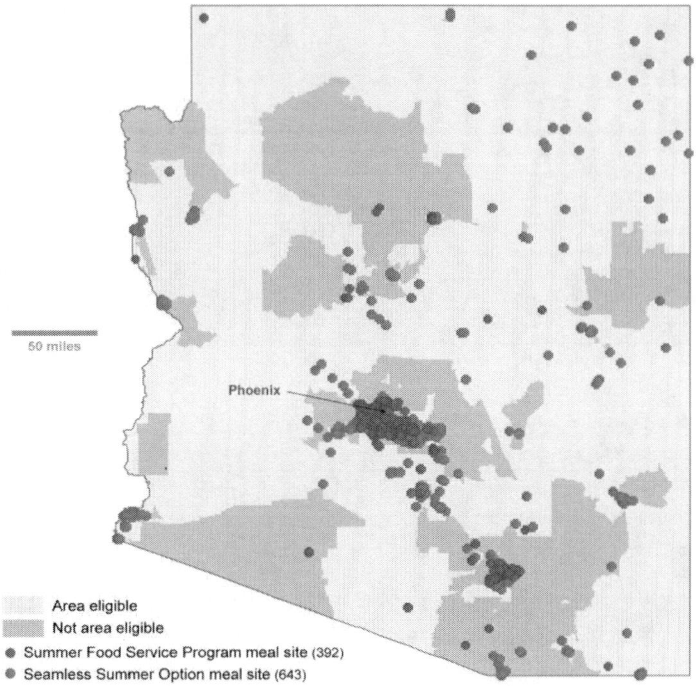

Source: GAO map based on fiscal year 2016 meal site data from Arizona on the Summer Food Service Program (SFSP) and the National School Lunch Program's Seamless Summer Option meal sites for the month with the greatest number of meals served in Arizona (June) and area eligibility data from the Census Bureau's American Community Survey provided by Food and Nutrition Service for fiscal year 2016. MapInfo (map). | GAO-18-369.

Note: This figure shows area eligibility as determined by the Food and Nutrition Service's Capacity Builder mapping tool, which is based on the U.S. Census Bureau's American Community Survey estimates of children eligible for free and reduced-price meals by Census block group and tract. However, states and sponsors may use other data to determine whether sites are "area eligible." In addition, certain types of sites may participate in the SFSP and Seamless Summer Option even if they are not area eligible.

Figure 10. Area Eligibility and Summer Meal Sites for the Month with the Greatest Number of Meals Served in Arizona, June 2016.

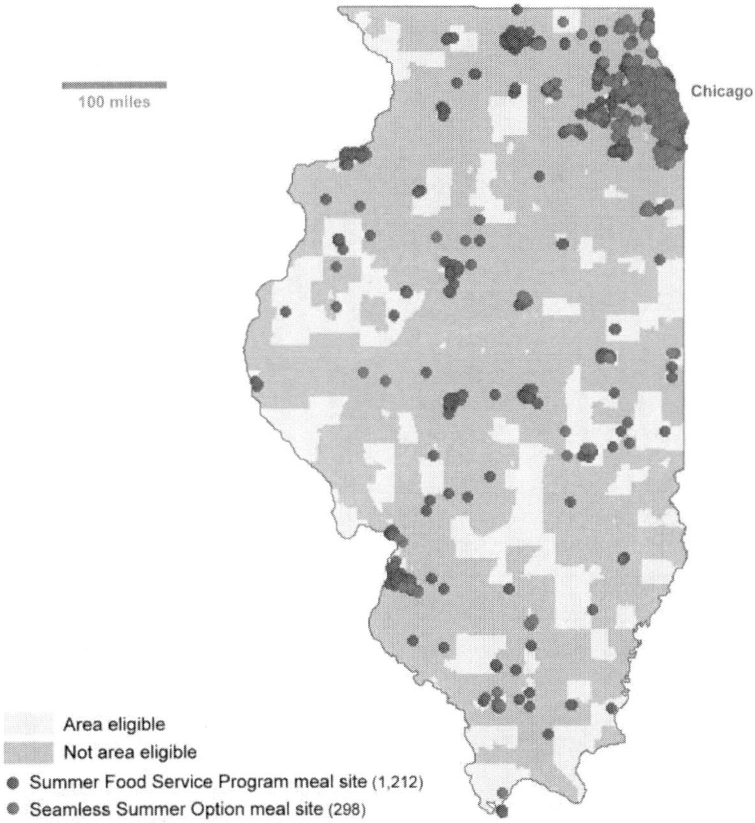

Source: GAO map based on fiscal year 2016 meal site data from Illinois on the Summer Food Service Program (SFSP) and the National School Lunch Program's Seamless Summer Option meal sites for the month with the greatest number of meals served in Illinois (July) and area eligibility data from the Census Bureau's American Community Survey provided by Food and Nutrition Service for fiscal year 2016. MapInfo (map). | GAO-18-369.

Note: This figure shows area eligibility as determined by the Food and Nutrition Service's Capacity Builder mapping tool, which is based on the U.S. Census Bureau's American Community Survey estimates of children eligible for free and reduced-price meals by Census block group and tract. However, states and sponsors may use other data to determine whether sites are "area eligible." In addition, certain types of sites may participate in the SFSP and Seamless Summer Option even if they are not area eligible.

Figure 11. Area Eligibility and Summer Meal Sites for the Month with the Greatest Number of Meals Served in Illinois, July 2016.

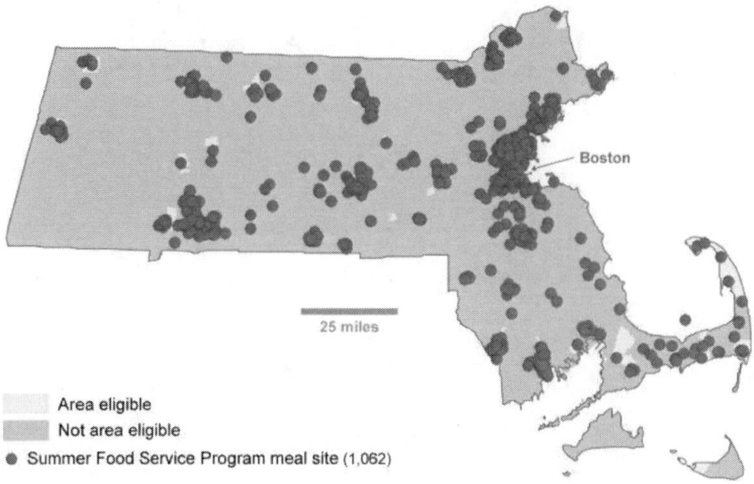

Source: GAO map based on fiscal year 2016 meal site data from Massachusetts on the Summer Food Service Program (SFSP) meal sites for the month with the greatest umber of meals served in Massachusetts (July) and area eligibility data from the Census Bureau's American Community Survey provided by Food and Nutrition Service for fiscal year 2016. MapInfo (map). | GAO-18-369.

Note: In summer 2016, Massachusetts had SFSP meal sites but no National School Lunch Program Seamless Summer Option sites. This figure shows area eligibility as determined by the Food and Nutrition Service's Capacity Builder mapping tool, which is based on the U.S. Census Bureau's American Community Survey estimates of children eligible for free and reduced-price meals by Census block group and tract. However, states and sponsors may use other data to determine whether sites are "area eligible." In addition, certain types of sites may participate in the SFSP and Seamless Summer Option even if they are not area eligible.

Figure 12. Area Eligibility and Summer Meal Sites for the Month with the Greatest Number of Meals Served in Massachusetts, July 2016.

In: Child Nutrition Programs
Editor: Daniel D. Coleman
ISBN: 978-1-53615-764-2

Chapter 5

SUMMER MEALS: IMPROVEMENTS NEEDED TO ADDRESS PARTICIPATION ESTIMATES AND PROGRAM CHALLENGES*

Kathryn A. Larin

Chairman Rokita, Ranking Member Polis, and Members of the Subcommittee:

I am pleased to be here today to discuss the U.S. Department of Agriculture's (USDA) Summer Food Service Program (SFSP). A federal nutrition program created in 1968, SFSP is designed to provide food service to children in low-income areas during periods when area schools are closed for vacation.[1] In fiscal year 2017, USDA spent $485 million to provide 152 million meals to children through the SFSP.

---

* This is an edited, reformatted and augmented version of United States Government Accountability Office; Testimony Before the Subcommittee on Early Childhood, Elementary, and Secondary Education, Committee on Education and the Workforce, House of Representatives; Accessible Version, Publication No. GAO-18-611T, dated July 17, 2018.

[1] See 42 U.S.C. § 1761. Children age 18 and under are eligible to participate. Eligible children also include individuals over age 18 who are determined by a state educational agency or a

USDA's Food and Nutrition Service (FNS) oversees the SFSP, which is administered by the states and operated by a variety of public and private nonprofit organizations and government entities that sponsor meals for children at supervised sites such as schools, camps, parks, churches, and libraries. FNS is responsible for issuing regulations,[2] instructions, and guidance; overseeing program administration; and reimbursing states for meals served that meet program requirements.[3] State agencies are responsible for approving and monitoring sponsors who, in turn, are responsible for monitoring and managing their meal sites.

SFSP meals must meet certain requirements in order to be eligible for federal reimbursement; for example, the meal must be served and consumed on-site at an approved meal site.[4] States may approve different types of meal sites, including open sites, closed enrolled sites, and camps. For example, open sites operate in an area where at least half of the children are eligible for free or reduced-price school meals (referred to as "area eligible"), according to data from entities such as schools or the U.S. Census Bureau.[5] Meals must also meet federal requirements for menu components, meal times, and nutrition.[6]

Some flexibilities are available to FNS in implementing the SFSP program, under its waiver and demonstration authorities. For example, the Secretary of Agriculture has statutory authority to waive, upon request of a state or eligible service provider, certain child nutrition program

---

local public educational agency of a state to have a disability, and who are participating in a public or nonprofit private school program established for individuals who have a disability.

[2] The SFSP program regulations are found at 7 C.F.R. pt. 225. Revisions to these regulations are scheduled to take effect July 31, 2018. This statement refers to the earlier version of the regulations, which were in effect at the time we did our work.

[3] States, in turn, provide funds to sponsors. Federal funding is also provided for certain SFSP administrative and operating costs.

[4] Specifically, program regulations require sponsors to maintain children on site while meals are consumed. 7 C.F.R. § 225.6(e)(15). This requirement, sometimes referred to as the "congregate meal requirement," is referred to as the "on-site requirement" throughout this statement.

[5] Children are generally eligible for free or reduced-priced school meals if their households have incomes at or below 185 percent of federal poverty guidelines. For example, see Child Nutrition Programs: Income Eligibility Guidelines, 82 Fed. Reg. 17, 182 (Apr.10, 2017).

[6] See 7 C.F.R. § 225.16.

requirements, including some for the SFSP.[7] To grant a waiver request, the Secretary must determine that the waiver would facilitate the state or service provider's ability to carry out the purpose of the program, and that the waiver will not increase the overall cost of the program to the federal government, among other things. In the event a waiver request is submitted, the Secretary is required to act promptly and state in writing whether the waiver request is granted or denied, and why. The Secretary is also required to periodically review the performance of waiver recipients, and submit an annual report to Congress summarizing the use of waivers and their effectiveness, among other details.[8]

In addition to this waiver authority, the Secretary is also authorized to carry out demonstration projects to develop and test methods of providing access to summer meals for low-income children in urban and rural areas, to reduce or eliminate the food insecurity and hunger of low-income children and improve their nutritional status.[9] The Secretary is required to provide for an independent evaluation of the demonstration projects carried out under this authority, and submit an annual report to Congress on the status of each project and the results of the evaluations.[10]

---

[7] 42 U.S.C. § 1760(l). Eligible service providers include SFSP sponsors. This waiver authority is subject to specified exceptions; for example, the Secretary may not grant waivers that relate to the nutritional content of meals served or federal reimbursement rates, among other things.

[8] The Secretary is required to annually submit to the Committee on Education and Labor of the House of Representatives and the Committee on Agriculture, Nutrition, and Forestry of the Senate a report that summarizes the use of waivers by the state and eligible service providers; describes whether the waivers resulted in improved services to children; describes the impact of the waivers on providing nutritional meals to participants; and describes how the waivers reduced the quantity of paperwork necessary to administer the program.

[9] This demonstration authority was first established and funded by the Agriculture, Rural Development, Food and Drug Administration, and Related Agencies Appropriations Act, 2010, Pub. L. No. 111-80, § 749(g), 123 Stat. 2090, 2132-33. Subsequent appropriations acts continued to fund these demonstrations, most recently the Consolidated Appropriations Act, 2018, Pub. L. No. 115-141, div. A, tit. IV, 132 Stat. 348.

[10] Each December 31, the Secretary is required to submit a report to the Committee on Education and Labor of the House of Representatives and the Committee on Agriculture, Nutrition, and Forestry of the Senate that includes the status of each demonstration project and the results of the evaluations for the previous fiscal year. Further, not later than 120 days after the completion of the last evaluation, the Secretary is required to submit a report to the same committees that includes recommendations to improve children's access to food during the summer months when school is not in regular session.

My testimony today summarizes the findings from our May 2018 report on summer meals.[11] This statement addresses (1) what is known about SFSP participation, (2) other programs that help feed low-income children over the summer, and (3) challenges in providing summer meals to children and the extent to which USDA provides assistance to address these challenges. To address these objectives, we reviewed relevant federal laws, regulations, and guidance; analyzed USDA's SFSP data for fiscal years 2007 through 2016; and surveyed state agencies responsible for administering the SFSP in 50 states and the District of Columbia. We also visited a nongeneralizable group of 3 states and 30 meal sites, selected based on Census data on child poverty rates and urban and rural locations, and analyzed meal site data from these 3 states. In addition, we interviewed USDA, state, and national organization officials, as well as SFSP providers, including sponsors and site operators. Our work was performed in accordance with generally accepted government auditing standards. More details on our scope and methodology can be found in the issued report.

In brief, we found that although USDA collects information about the actual number of meals served to children through the SFSP program—which is one indicator of program participation—USDA's estimates of the number of children participating in the SFSP were unreliable. As a result, USDA's understanding of children's participation in the SFSP was limited, impairing its ability to both inform program implementation and facilitate strategic planning and outreach to areas with low participation.

Other federal and nonfederal programs helped feed low-income children over the summer to some extent. These federal programs included the National School Lunch Program's Seamless Summer Option, which provides nutrition assistance benefits solely in the summer, and several federal programs that operate year-round. Nonfederal programs, commonly operated by local faith-based organizations and foodbanks, also helped feed low-income children in the summer, but states and local organizations reported that these had limited reach.

---

[11] GAO, *Summer Meals: Actions Needed to Improve Participation Estimates and Address Program Challenges*, GAO-18-369 (Washington, D.C.: May 31, 2018).

Finally, there were gaps in USDA's efforts to address reported challenges related to SFSP meal site safety and program administration. Although USDA had granted some states and sponsors flexibility from the requirement that children consume meals on-site when safety at the site was a concern, the agency did not broadly communicate the circumstances it considers when granting this flexibility, hindering its usefulness in ensuring safe summer meal delivery to children. Additionally, while FNS had established program and policy simplifications to help lessen the administrative burden on sponsors participating in multiple child nutrition programs, challenges in this area persisted. Some of these simplifications had not been shared recently with states, potentially discouraging sponsor participation in child nutrition programs and limiting children's access to meals.

My statement will highlight four recommendations we made in our May report that USDA should implement to help improve SFSP participation estimates and address challenges reported by states and sponsors related to meal site safety and duplicative paperwork. In oral comments, FNS officials, including the Deputy Administrator for Child Nutrition Programs, generally agreed with the recommendations in the report.

THE NUMBER OF SFSP MEALS SERVED GENERALLY INCREASED FROM 2007 THROUGH 2016, BUT ESTIMATES OF CHILDREN PARTICIPATING WERE UNRELIABLE

The total number of SFSP meals served nationwide during the summer— one indicator of program participation—increased from 113 million meals in fiscal year 2007 to 149 million meals in fiscal year 2016, or by 32 percent.[12] Although almost half of the total increase in meals

[12] Trends in meals served nationwide were based on our analysis of FNS data, which we determined were sufficiently reliable for the purposes of our May 2018 report. Unless otherwise noted, our report focused on SFSP meals served during the summer months, which we defined to include May, June, July, and August. Nationwide refers to the 50 states

served in the summer months was due to increases in lunches, when comparing across each of the meal types, supper and breakfast had the largest percentage increases over the 10-year period, 50 and 48 percent, respectively (see Table 1).[13] The increase in SFSP meals over this time period was generally consistent with increases in the number of meals served in the National School Lunch Program (NSLP), the largest child nutrition assistance program, during this period.

Table 1. Change in Number of Meals Served Nationwide in the Food and Nutrition Service's Summer Food Service Program (SFSP) by Meal Type, Fiscal Years 2007 and 2016

n/a	Number of SFSP Meals Served by Meal Service Type				
n/a	Breakfast	Lunch	Supper	Snack	Total
2007 (fiscal year)	28,512,170	68,085,416	4,166,516	12,210,737	112,974,839
2016 (fiscal year)	42,329,229	85,708,601	6,254,579	14,868,097	149,160,506
Increase in number of meals serviced	13,817,059	17,623,185	2,088,063	2,657,360	36,185,667
Percent increase	48	26	50	22	N/A

Legend: n/a = not applicable.

Source: GAO analysis of data provided by the Food and Nutrition Service. I GAO-18-369.

Note: SFSP meals served include breakfast, lunch, supper, and snack. This figure includes meals served in the 50 states and the District of Columbia during May, June, July, and August. Our review focused on changes in the 10 years from fiscal year 2007 through fiscal year 2016.

Although states reported the actual number of SFSP meals served to FNS for reimbursement purposes, they *estimated* the number of children participating in SFSP, and these participation estimates have been calculated inconsistently, impairing FNS's ability to inform program implementation and facilitate strategic planning and outreach to areas with

---

and the District of Columbia. The SFSP primarily operates during school vacation from May through September (accounting for more than 99 percent of meals served in fiscal year 2016), but it also operates during vacation periods in any month for programs operating on continuous school calendars, and during certain other times for areas affected by unanticipated school closure, such as for a natural disaster. In addition, our review focused on fiscal year 2007 through fiscal year 2016, and included all SFSP meals served: breakfast, lunch, supper, and snack.

[13] For example, suppers increased from 4,166,516 meals served in 2007 to 6,254,579 meals served in 2016. Breakfasts increased from 28,512,170 meals served in 2007 to 42,329,229 meals served in 2016.

low participation. Specifically, state agencies calculated a statewide estimate of children's participation in the SFSP, referred to as average daily attendance (ADA), using sponsor-reported information on the number of meals served and days of operation in July of each year.[14] However, according to our review of states' survey responses and FNS documents, states' methods for calculating ADA have differed from state to state and from year to year. For example, although FNS directed states to include the number of meals served in each site's primary meal service—which may or may not be lunch—some states calculated ADA using only meals served at lunch. In addition, five states reported in our survey that the method they used to calculate ADA in fiscal year 2016 differed from the one they used previously.[15]

While FNS clarified its instructions in May 2017 to help improve the consistency of states' ADA calculations moving forward, ADA, even if consistently calculated, remained an unreliable estimate of children's daily participation in SFSP for at least two reasons. First, ADA did not account for existing variation in the number of days that each site serves meals to children. Specifically, because FNS's instructions indicated that sites' ADAs were to be combined to provide a statewide ADA estimate, differences in the number of days of meal service at each site were disregarded. As a result, ADA did not reflect the average number of children served SFSP meals daily throughout the month.[16] Second, ADA was an unreliable estimate of children's participation in SFSP because it

---

[14] States report this information to FNS on Form FNS-418: Report of the Summer Food Service Program for Children. Sponsors first report to states a total average daily attendance (ADA) across all of their sites, which is calculated by dividing the number of meals served at each site's primary meal service by the number of days each site operated in July, the month FNS has determined most SFSP meals are served, according to FNS officials. States combine sponsor ADAs for a statewide ADA for July. FNS combines states' ADAs to estimate children's participation in the SFSP nationwide.

[15] Seven additional states reported that they were unsure if they had changed the method used to calculate ADA in fiscal year 2016.

[16] For example, according to data provided by one selected state, three sites in that state had a reported ADA of 60 for July. Yet two of the sites served meals to children on only 1 day of the month and the other site served meals to children on 20 days. Although 120 children were served SFSP meals only 1 day in July across two of these sites, the combined ADA across all three sites, which we calculated following FNS's instructions, inaccurately suggests an average of 180 children were participating in SFSP at these sites on a daily basis in July.

did not account for state variation in the month with the greatest number of SFSP meals served. According to FNS officials, the agency instructed states to calculate ADA for July because officials identified this as the month with the largest number of meals served nationwide. However, according to our analysis of nationwide FNS data, in summer 2016, 26 states served more SFSP meals in June or August than in July.[17]

Although FNS had taken some steps to identify other data that states collect on the SFSP, at the time of our May 2018 report, FNS had not yet used this information to help improve its estimate of children's participation in the program. In 2015, FNS published a Request for Information, asking whether states or sponsors collected any SFSP data that were not reported to FNS, and received responses from 15 states.[18] The responses suggested some states collected additional data, such as site-level data, that may allow for an improved estimate of children's SFSP participation, potentially addressing the issues identified in our analysis. FNS also followed up with several of these states in 2016 and 2017 to explore the feasibility of collecting additional data and improving estimates of children's SFSP participation.[19] FNS stated in a May 2017 memo to states that it is critical that the agency's means of estimating children's participation in the SFSP is as accurate as possible because it helps inform program implementation at the national level and facilitates

[17] For example, for one selected state, Arizona, we followed FNS's instructions and found that using July to calculate ADA cut the participation estimate almost in half—14,987 in July 2016 compared to 26,772 in June 2016. State officials in Arizona explained that schools typically end the academic year in May and return to school in July, therefore, June is the busiest month for SFSP in Arizona.

[18] Request for Information: Summer Meal Programs Data Reporting Requirements, 80 Fed. Reg. 12,423 (March. 9, 2015).

[19] Although they took these steps, FNS officials told us they were cognizant of the burden on states and site operators that would be associated with additional reporting requirements. FNS officials indicated they were conducting a study related to child nutrition program reporting requirements, as required by the Consolidated Appropriations Act, 2017. See Pub. L. No. 115-31, div. A, tit. I, 131 Stat. 135, 161. FNS officials said they expected the study to be completed in November 2018. They noted that some states expressed concerns in the ongoing study about the burden of child nutrition reporting requirements. Further, FNS officials noted that collection of additional information from states would require OMB approval under the Paperwork Reduction Act, and may also require regulatory changes.

strategic planning and outreach to areas with low participation.[20] Yet, at the time of our report, FNS had not taken further action to improve the estimate. In our May 2018 report, we concluded that FNS's limited understanding of children's participation in the SFSP impaired its ability to both inform program implementation and facilitate strategic planning and outreach to areas with low participation.

To improve FNS's estimate of children's participation in the SFSP, we recommended that FNS focus on addressing, at a minimum, data reliability issues caused by variations in the number of operating days of meal sites and in the months in which states see the greatest number of meals served. FNS generally agreed with this recommendation.

Other Federal and Nonfederal Programs Helped Feed Low-Income Children over the Summer to Some Extent

Other federal and nonfederal programs that operate solely in the summer, as well as those operating year-round, helped feed low-income children in the summer months. For example, in 2016, FNS data indicated about 26 million meals were served through the NSLP's Seamless Summer Option, a separate federal program that streamlines administrative requirements for school meal providers serving summer meals.[21] Some children also received summer meals through nonfederal programs operated by entities such as faith-based organizations and foodbanks, though the reach of these efforts was limited, according to our state survey and interviews with providers and national organizations at the time of our report. For example, of the 27 states that reported in our survey awareness of the geographic coverage of these nonfederal programs, 11 states

[20] USDA, Food and Nutrition Service, *Revisions to Instructions for the Calculation for Average Daily Attendance on the Form FNS-418*, Memo code SFSP 09-2017 (Alexandria, VA: May 10, 2017).

[21] These data included meals provided in the 50 states and the District of Columbia. For more information about FNS's estimates, see GAO-18-369.

indicated that they operated in some portions of the state—the most common state response.[22]

STATES AND SFSP PROVIDERS FACED CHALLENGES WITH MEAL SITES, PARTICIPATION, AND PROGRAM ADMINISTRATION, AND FNS ACTIONS HAD ADDRESSED SOME, BUT NOT ALL AREAS

States and SFSP providers reported challenges with issues related to meal site availability, children's participation, and program administration, though federal, state, and local entities had taken steps to improve these areas. For example, a lack of available transportation, low population density, and limited meal sites posed challenges for SFSP implementation in rural areas, according to states we surveyed, selected national organizations, and state and local officials in the three states we visited. In response, state and local entities took steps, such as transporting meals to children by bus, to address these issues—efforts that FNS supported through information sharing and grants.

States and SFSP providers also reported challenges with meal site safety, and FNS's efforts to address this area were limited. Seventeen states reported in our survey that ensuring summer meal sites are in safe locations was moderately to very challenging.[23] Some states and sponsors took steps to help address this issue, and FNS also used its available authorities to grant some states and sponsors flexibility with respect to the requirement that children consume summer meals on site, such as when

[22] In addition, 16 states reported that they were not aware of any nonfederal programs providing summer meals to children in their state, 7 states reported that they did not know, and 1 state did not respond.

[23] In addition to the 17 states that reported on the issue of safe locations as moderately to very challenging, 14 states reported this issue as slightly challenging, 7 states reported this as not at all challenging, 3 states reported they did not know, and 10 states reported no response. In our survey, we did not define "safe locations." For more information on our survey results and the full list of challenges states reported, see appendix II in GAO-18-369.

safety at the site is a concern. However, our review of FNS documentation showed FNS had not clearly communicated to all states and sponsors the circumstances it considers when deciding whether to grant this flexibility.[24] These circumstances—described in letters the agency sent to requesting states—generally included verification that violent crime activities occurred within both a 6-block radius of the meal site and 72 hours prior to the meal service.[25] Although FNS officials explained that they reviewed state and sponsor requests for flexibility due to safety concerns on a case-by-case basis, they also acknowledged that the set of circumstances they used to approve state and sponsor requests for flexibility, which we identified in their letters to states, had been used repeatedly. Further, states and sponsors reported challenges obtaining the specific data needed for approval of a site for this type of flexibility, including inconsistent availability of timely data, which hampered some providers' efforts to ensure safe delivery of meals.

We concluded that unless FNS shared information with all states and sponsors on the circumstances it considered when deciding whether to grant flexibility with respect to the requirement that children consume summer meals on site, states and sponsors would likely continue to be challenged to use this flexibility, hindering its usefulness in ensuring safe summer meal delivery to children. We therefore recommended that FNS communicate to all SFSP stakeholders the circumstances it considers in approving requests for flexibility with respect to the requirement that children consume SFSP meals on-site in areas that have experienced crime and violence, taking into account the feasibility of accessing data needed

---

[24] Although FNS had issued guidance on the general processes for requesting flexibility from program requirements under its waiver and demonstration authorities, these guidance documents did not detail the specific circumstances that the agency considered when deciding whether to grant flexibility from the on-site requirement due to safety concerns. For more information about FNS's guidance, see GAO-18-369 and FNS's policy memos SP 14-2017, SFSP 07-2017, Demonstration Project for Non-Congregate Feeding for Outdoor Summer Meal Sites Experiencing Excessive Heat with Q&As (January 2017), and SP 27-2017, CACFP 12-2017, SFSP 08-2017, Child Nutrition Program Waiver Request Guidance and Protocol (April 2017).

[25] Violent crime activities were defined in FNS's letters to states as murder, attempted murder, aggravated assault, and armed robbery.

for approval, to ensure safe delivery of meals to children. FNS generally agreed with this recommendation.

We also found that while FNS had issued reports to Congress evaluating some of its demonstration projects, as required under its statutory authorities, the agency had not issued any such reports to Congress specifically on the use of flexibilities with respect to the on-site requirement in areas where safety was a concern. As previously discussed, the agency is required to annually submit certain reports to Congress regarding the use of waivers and evaluations of projects carried out under its demonstration authority.[26] FNS officials told us that they had not evaluated or reported on these flexibilities, in part, because they had limited information on their outcomes.[27]

We concluded that without understanding the impact of its use of these flexibilities, neither FNS nor Congress knew whether these flexibilities were helping provide meals to children—the goal of the program. Accordingly, we recommended that FNS evaluate and annually report to Congress, as required by statute, on its use of waivers and demonstration projects to grant states and sponsors flexibility with respect to the requirement that children consume SFSP meals on-site in areas experiencing crime or violence, to improve understanding of the use and

---

[26] The Secretary of Agriculture is required to annually submit to the Committee on Education and Labor in the House of Representatives and the Committee on Agriculture, Nutrition, and Forestry of the Senate a report that summarizes the use of waivers and describes whether they resulted in improved services to children, the impact of the waivers on providing nutritional meals to participants, and how the waivers reduced the quantity of paperwork necessary to administer the program. 42 U.S.C. § 1760(l). In addition, the Secretary is required to provide for an independent evaluation of the projects carried out under its demonstration authority, and submit annual reports to the same Committees on the status of each demonstration project and the results of the evaluations for the previous fiscal year. Further, not later than 120 days after the completion of the last evaluation, the Secretary is required to submit a report that includes recommendations on how to improve children's access to food during the summer months when school is not in regular session. See the Agriculture, Rural Development, Food and Drug Administration, and Related Agencies Appropriations Act, 2010, Pub. L. No. 111-80, § 749(g), 123 Stat. 2090, 2132-33, most recently funded by the Consolidated Appropriations Act, 2018, Pub. L. No. 115-141, div. A, tit. IV, 132 Stat. 348.

[27] In its letters to states approving their requests for flexibility with the requirement to consume meals on-site when safety is a concern, FNS asked states and sponsors to submit reports on the implementation and results of the flexibility. However, FNS officials told us they did not always receive this information.

impact of granting these flexibilities on meeting program goals. FNS generally agreed with this recommendation.

Although FNS had established program and policy simplifications to help lessen the administrative burden on sponsors participating in multiple child nutrition programs, challenges in this area persisted, indicating that information had not reached all relevant state agencies. According to officials we spoke with from a national organization involved in summer meals, management of each child nutrition program and the processes related to applications, funding, and oversight were fragmented in many states. For example, in one of the states we visited, a sponsor that provided school meals during the school year told us they had to fill out 60 additional pages of paperwork to provide summer meals, which they described as significant burden. FNS officials told us that some of the duplicative requirements might have been a function of differences in statute, and although FNS provided guidance to states on simplified procedures for sponsors participating in more than one child nutrition program, some states might have chosen not to implement them.

We concluded that without further efforts from FNS to disseminate information on current options for streamlining administrative requirements across multiple child nutrition programs, overlapping and duplicative administrative requirements may limit children's access to meals by discouraging sponsor participation in child nutrition programs. We recommended that FNS disseminate information about the existing streamlining options, and FNS generally agreed with this recommendation.

Chairman Rokita, Ranking Member Polis, and Members of the Subcommittee, this concludes my prepared statement. I would be pleased to respond to any questions you may have at this time.

In: Child Nutrition Programs
Editor: Daniel D. Coleman
ISBN: 978-1-53615-764-2

Chapter 6

A PRIMER ON WIC: THE SPECIAL SUPPLEMENTAL NUTRITION PROGRAM FOR WOMEN, INFANTS, AND CHILDREN (UPDATED)*

Randy Alison Aussenberg

ABSTRACT

The Special Supplemental Nutrition Program for Women, Infants, and Children (WIC) provides nutrition-rich foods, nutrition education (including breastfeeding promotion and support), and health care and social services referrals to eligible low-income women, infants, and children. In FY2016, approximately 7.7 million people participated in WIC each month. WIC is authorized by the Child Nutrition Act, as is the related WIC Farmers' Market Nutrition Program (WIC FMNP). WIC, WIC FMNP, school meals, and the other child nutrition programs are typically reauthorized together; these programs were last reauthorized in the Healthy, Hunger-Free Kids Act of 2010 (P.L. 111-296).

* This is an edited, reformatted and augmented version of Congressional Research Service, Publication No. R44115, dated April 7, 2017.

WIC's funding is discretionary, and the bulk of program funds are allocated via formula grant to state agencies for food costs and "Nutrition Services and Administration." In FY2016, there were 90 state agencies (50 states, District of Columbia, 5 U.S. territories, and 34 Indian Tribal Organizations). These agencies operate the program through local WIC agencies and clinics. The program obligated over $7 billion in federal funds in FY2014.

WIC has a number of federal and state eligibility rules, including categorical, financial, and nutritional risk. Participants must fall into one of WIC's participant categories: pregnant, postpartum, and breastfeeding women; infants; or children (under five years of age). Financial eligibility is met if (1) a household has income at or below 185% of the federal poverty level, or (2) applicants receive benefits through Temporary Assistance for Needy Families (TANF), the Supplemental Nutrition Assistance Program (SNAP), Medicaid, or certain state programs. Households also must meet nutritional risk criteria and reside in the state of application.

WIC provides participants with monthly benefits redeemable for specified foods to supplement their diets, as well as related nutrition and health services. WIC-eligible foods are laid out in federal regulation, and state agencies develop their own approved food lists within this framework. At the WIC clinic, participants are provided the benefits to redeem specific foods (food package) for the participant's category and individual nutritional needs. Major changes to the federal WIC food package regulations have been made in recent years; for some participant categories, the food package now includes a cash-value voucher redeemable for fruits and vegetables. One way that state agencies control WIC costs is through their approved foods lists. These lists usually include one brand of infant formula, as state agencies are required to control infant formula costs through competitive bidding for infant formula rebate contracts. In addition to providing food benefits, states are required to ensure that nutrition education, including breastfeeding promotion and drug abuse education, is available to all pregnant, postpartum, and breastfeeding participants in the program. Agencies also work to refer WIC participants to health services and other public programs, particularly Medicaid.

Nearly all states administer their programs through a retail food delivery system, in which participants purchase foods at authorized retailers (vendors). Accordingly, many WIC policies at the federal and state levels pertain to vendor authorization and oversight as well as benefit redemption. Currently, most states distribute checks or vouchers for participants to purchase WIC foods at vendors; however, state agencies are increasingly transitioning to electronic benefit transfer (EBT), in part because the 2010 reauthorization law requires this transition by October 1, 2020. States authorize vendors for the program, considering factors like a vendor's inventory and capacity and geographic distribution of vendors. States also consider and monitor WIC vendors' pricing, as required by federal law, to help contain program costs.

INTRODUCTION AND BACKGROUND

The Special Supplemental Nutrition Program for Women, Infants, and Children (WIC) provides supplemental nutrition-rich foods and nutrition education (including breastfeeding promotion and support), as well as referrals to health care and social services, to low-income, nutritionally at-risk women, infants, and children up to five years old. Eligible women are specifically limited to those pregnant and postpartum (if breastfeeding, women are eligible for more benefits for a longer period of time). The WIC program seeks to improve the health status of its participants and prevent the occurrence of health problems during critical times of growth and development.[1]

WIC is a federally funded program administered by the U.S. Department of Agriculture's Food and Nutrition Service (USDA-FNS). In FY2016, approximately 7.7 million people participated in WIC each month in programs run by 90 state agencies (50 states, District of Columbia, 5 U.S. territories, and 34 Indian Tribal Organizations).[2] USDA has said roughly half of all infants in the United States participate in the WIC program.[3]

This chapter provides an overview of the WIC program, including administration, funding, eligibility, benefits, benefits redemption, and cost containment policies. While this chapter is meant to be a primer and is not focused on tracking major policy issues, it may be useful for the reader to note that this chapter does discuss features of the WIC program that are

---

[1] See Section 17(a) of the Child Nutrition Act (codified at 42 U.S.C. 1786(a)) for program declaration of purpose. Subsequent citations to WIC's authorizing statute will list only the U.S. Code citation.

[2] WIC Program Participation and Costs, available at USDA-FNS website, https://www.fns.usda.gov/pd/wic-program.

[3] See USDA-FNS website, "About WIC- WIC at a Glance," http://www.fns.usda.gov/wic/about-wic-wic-glance.

often the topic of policy debate: funding, eligible foods, and the redemption of benefits.

Authorization and Reauthorization

The WIC program dates back to a 1972 amendment to the Child Nutrition Act, which created WIC as a two-year pilot program. WIC became a permanent program in 1975 and remains authorized by Section 17 of the Child Nutrition Act (codified at 42 U.S.C. 1786). Congressional jurisdiction over this law has typically been exercised by the Senate Committee on Agriculture, Nutrition, and Forestry and the House Committee on Education and the Workforce.

Congress periodically reviews and reauthorizes expiring authorities under the Child Nutrition Act, generally in conjunction with the "Child Nutrition Programs,"[4] which are authorized by the Richard B. Russell National School Lunch Act, Section 32 of the Act of August 24, 1935, and the Child Nutrition Act.[5] WIC and the Child Nutrition Programs were most recently reauthorized in 2010 through the Healthy, Hunger-Free Kids Act of 2010 (HHFKA, P.L. 111-296), and those authorities that expire do so after September 30, 2015 (the end of FY2015). During the 114th Congress, committees of jurisdiction marked up bills to reauthorize WIC but reauthorization was not completed. As of the date of this chapter, no bills to reauthorize WIC have been introduced or marked up in the 115th Congress.

The WIC Farmers' Market Nutrition Program (WIC FMNP) is closely related to WIC and also authorized within Section 17 of the Child Nutrition Act (Section 17(m)). This program, which serves much of WIC's population, is also typically reauthorized during the reauthorization of WIC and the Child Nutrition Program. This chapter discusses WIC and not WIC

---

[4] "Child Nutrition Programs" is a category used to describe USDA-FNS programs that help to provide food for children in school or institutional settings.

[5] For an overview of federal child nutrition programs typically reauthorized with WIC, see CRS Report R43783, *School Meals Programs and Other USDA Child Nutrition Programs: A Primer*.

FMNP; however, a brief overview of that program is provided in Appendix C.

Federal, State, and Local Administration

WIC operates through a federal, state, and local partnership. The U.S. Department of Agriculture's Food and Nutrition Service (USDA-FNS) administers the WIC program at the federal level. USDA-FNS provides cash grants for foods and "Nutrition Services and Administration" to 90 state agencies (50 states, District of Columbia, 5 U.S. territories, and 34 Indian Tribal Organizations), which operate the program through local WIC agencies and clinics.[6]

At the federal level, USDA-FNS is responsible for issuing and enforcing regulations, providing technical assistance to state agencies, and conducting studies and producing reports to evaluate the WIC program.[7] At the state level, state agencies are generally responsible for program operations within their jurisdictions. States provide subgrants and technical assistance to local WIC agencies. Federal law and regulations allow states some flexibility in program operations, including options for food delivery systems and benefit redemption systems.[8] States also have discretion in deciding the specific brands, types, and package sizes to include in their approved WIC food packages, within the bounds of federal regulations.[9] At the local level, local WIC agencies—generally state and county health departments—provide WIC services and benefits directly or through local

---

[6] 42 U.S.C. 1786(c). NOTE: Since 2000, the Department of Defense (DOD) administers a similar program known as the WIC Overseas Program. The program is available to eligible participants living overseas, including civilian employees, Department of Defense contractors, members of the uniformed service and their family members. Established under 10 U.S.C. 1060a(a), the program is administered by DOD, not USDA, and is paid for with DOD funds. Further information can be found on Tricare's website: http://www.tricare.mil/wic/. This CRS report will not discuss the DOD program and data cited within does not include it.

[7] 42 U.S.C. 1786(g)(5).

[8] See "Redemption of Food Benefits and Related Cost Containment Policies" section of this chapter for more information on food delivery systems.

[9] 7 C.F.R. 246.10.

service sites and clinics. As of February 2015, there are approximately 1,900 local WIC agencies operating the program in approximately 10,000 local service sites or clinics.[10]

Funding

Funding for WIC food and services is primarily provided by the federal government; though some states supplement their programs with their own funding, WIC law does not require matching funds. WIC's funding is categorized as discretionary with funding amounts determined entirely through the annual appropriations process.[11] Since the late 1990s, the appropriations committees' practice has been to provide enough funds for WIC to serve all eligible applicants who seek program benefits (i.e., all forecasted participants).[12]

Table 1. WIC Appropriations, FY2012-FY2016
In millions of dollars

	FY2012 (P.L. 112-55)	FY2013 (P.L. 113-6)[a]	FY2014 (P.L. 113-76)	FY2015 (P.L. 113- 235)	FY2016 (P.L. 114-113)
WIC Account					
Total	$6,618.5	$6,522.2	$6,715.8	$6,623.0	$6,350.0[b]

Source: CRS, compiled from respective appropriations laws and related congressional documents.

[a] This funding level displayed is post-sequester. For more information on the FY2013 sequester of funds provided by the Agriculture and Related Agencies appropriations bill, based on the Budget Control Act of 2011, see CRS Report R43110, *Agriculture and Related Agencies: FY2014 and FY2013 (Post-Sequestration) Appropriations*.

[b] In addition, Section 751 provided $220 million for management information systems and WIC EBT by rescinding FY2015 carryover and recovery funding.

---

[10] See USDA-FNS website, "About WIC-WIC at a Glance," http://www.fns.usda.gov/wic/about-wic-wic-glance.

[11] A minor exception, 42 U.S.C. 1786(h)(13) directly appropriates $1 million per year for a Universal Product Code (UPC) database. This funding is mandatory.

[12] "Anecdotal evidence suggest that WIC became fully funded sometime in the late 1990s," Victor Oliveira and Elizabeth Frazão, *The WIC Program: Background, Trends, and Economic Issues, 2015 Edition*, EIB-134, U.S. Department of Agriculture, Economic Research Service, January 2015, p.19. (Hereinafter cited as "Oliveira and Frazão, EIB-134 (2015)").

Lower levels of funding for the WIC program could reduce the number of pregnant and postpartum women, infants, and children served. The WIC program is typically funded through the annual Agriculture and Related Agencies appropriations bill. Funds are available for two years (e.g., FY2015 appropriations are available for obligation through FY2016). Table 1 displays the funding provided for the WIC account in recent years' appropriations laws.

The majority of WIC's funding is distributed by USDA-FNS to states based upon allocation formulas described in federal regulations.[13] The formulas used to allocate federal funds—both money from the annual appropriation and any unused money recovered and reallocated—are designed to (1) guarantee states enough money to maintain their previous year's operating level and caseload (with adjustments for inflation), and (2) distribute any extra dollars to grantees receiving comparatively less than their "fair share" of funds (based on their income-eligible WIC population and amount estimated as needed to serve their projected participation level).[14] As needed and authorized, USDA-FNS may reallocate funding throughout the year.[15] State-by-state allocation amounts for recent and past years can be found at USDA-FNS's website.[16]

In addition to the appropriated funding provided for the current fiscal year, WIC may carry over funds remaining from the prior year's appropriation; and in the event that these funds from two years prove insufficient, the program maintains a contingency fund that can be spent in any year.[17] Table 2 displays three years of federal WIC obligations. Due to the availability of WIC's appropriated funds, obligated funds may include not only the current year's appropriation but carryover and contingency spending as well.

---

[13] 7 C.F.R. 246.16.

[14] 7 C.F.R. 246.16(c)(2), (3). See also, Dawn K. Aldridge, "Special Supplemental Nutrition Program for Women, Infants, and Children (WIC) Funding Formula Evolution," *Journal of Official Statistics*, vol. 18, no. 3 (2002), pp. 430 433.

[15] 7 C.F.R. 246.16(c)-(e).

[16] http://www.fns.usda.gov/wic/wic-funding-and-program-data.

[17] After the contingency fund had been depleted, Congress provided $125 million funds to be held in contingency in the FY2014 appropriations law (P.L. 113-76).

Table 2. WIC Obligations, FY2012-FY2015
In millions of dollars

Project/Purpose	FY2012	FY2013	FY2014	FY2015
Grants to States:				
Supplemental Food	4,780	4,823	4,889	4,680
Nutrition Services and Administration	1,926	2,013	2,013	1,990
Subtotal, Grants to States	6,706	6,835	6,902	6,670
Infrastructure Grants	3	13	7	10
Technical Assistance	-	-	0[a]	0[a]
Breastfeeding Peer Counselors	60	55	60	60
Management Information Systems	10	32	36	10
Program Evaluation & Monitoring	10	5	8	13
Federal Administration	9	10	6	3
WIC Contingency Funds	368	-	125	0
UPC Database[b]	2	1	1	0[a]
TOTAL WIC FUNDS				
OBLIGATED	$7,168	$6,952	$7,145	$6,768

Sources: FY2012 data from FNS FY2015 Congressional Budget Justification (p. 32-63); FY2013, FY2014 data from FNS FY2016 Congressional Budget Justification (p. 32-67); FY2015 data from FNS FY2017 Congressional Budget Justification (p. 32-76).

Notes: Numbers may not add, due to rounding.

[a] Less than $1 million.

[b] Per Section 17(h)(13) of the Child Nutrition Act of 1966 (42 U.S.C. 1786(h)(13)), funding for this purpose is directly appropriated. This Universal Product Code (UPC) database supports states' transition to EBT.

As Table 2 shows, the bulk of WIC funding is provided as two types of grants for states: food grants, and Nutrition Services and Administration (NSA) grants. Food grant funds may be used to pay retail grocery stores for foods purchased by program participants; to acquire, store, and provide supplemental foods to participants; and to purchase or rent breast pumps.[18] NSA grant funds may be used for participant certification costs, nutrition education activities, breastfeeding promotion and support activities, and salaries and administrative costs to provide these services.[19] In general, money for food costs and NSA expenses must be kept separate; however, grantees may, under federal guidelines, convert food funding to support NSA costs. The WIC appropriation also includes federal funds for

[18] 7 C.F.R. 246.14(b).

[19] 42 U.S.C. 1786(a)(4), 7 C.F.R. 246.14(c).

specified WIC purposes (e.g., Management Information Systems, Breastfeeding Peer Counselors) that may only be used to carry out approved projects or certain activities.

Because WIC's funding is tied to the cost of food items, the program has come to include a number of cost containment measures. Such measures include approved food lists with reasonably priced food items, rebates on infant formula and other authorized foods, and the selection of WIC vendors based on competitive prices. These policies are discussed in later sections of this chapter.

ELIGIBILITY

Mothers and children seeking WIC assistance must apply to their local WIC agencies and be screened for eligibility.[20] WIC has a number of federal and state eligibility requirements including categorical, financial, and nutritional risk tests.[21]

Categorical Eligibility

To qualify for benefits, an individual must be categorically eligible (i.e., in a specified participant category).[22] WIC serves individuals in the following participant categories:

- women during pregnancy and up to six weeks after delivery,
- breastfeeding women up to one year after delivery,
- non-breastfeeding women up to six months postpartum,

---

[20] Physical presence of the applicant is required, unless a local agency determines that the physical presence of an applicant would present an unreasonable barrier to participation (42 U.S.C. 1786(d)(3)(C)).

[21] See generally 42 U.S.C. 1786(d).

[22] In the WIC program, "categorical eligibility" refers to the categories of individuals the program is designed to serve, different from the term in the Supplemental Nutrition Assistance Program (SNAP).

- infants, and
- children up to age five (eligibility ends at fifth birthday).

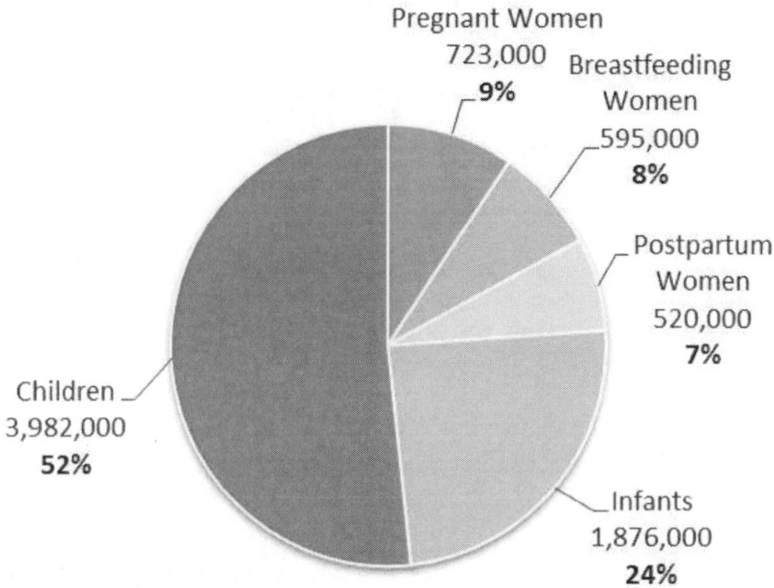

Source: Figure prepared by CRS using USDA-FNS Administrative Data. Rounded to the nearest thousand and nearest 1%.

Figure 1. WIC Participant Characteristics, by Category; FY2016, as of February 2017.

In FY2016, approximately 24% of participants were women, 24% were infants, and 52% were children under the age of 5.[23] Participant characteristics by category are shown in Figure 1.

Income Eligibility

Applicants must meet specific income guidelines to qualify for WIC, and applicants who participate in certain programs are deemed income-

[23] FNS Program Information Report, p. 30, http://www.fns.usda.gov/sites/default/files/datastatistics/keydata-september2016_0.pdf. For more information on monthly and state level data, see WIC Program Data, http://www.fns.usda.gov/ pd/wic-program.

eligible. Federal law states that the maximum allowable gross family income of an applicant must not exceed the guidelines for reduced-price school meals, which are set at 185% of the federal poverty level (income eligibility guidelines shown in Table 3).[24] Although federal regulation allows states to set income limits between 100% and 185% of the federal poverty level, currently all WIC state agencies set the income limit at the maximum of 185%. Federal law also sets the rules for what state agencies may exclude from counted income, with additional options provided in regulations.[25]

Applicants can become income-eligible for WIC by one of two pathways: (1) providing documentation of income below the 185% FPL threshold, or (2) being deemed eligible based on participation in certain means-tested programs (adjunctive eligibility).

In the first pathway, the income of the "family," not only the program participants, is considered. Federal regulation defines family largely as individuals (related or unrelated) who are living together.[26] State agencies have the option to choose the income time frame for applicants (e.g., annually or a shorter term).[27] WIC authorizing law includes state options for whether to count or exclude certain types of military income,[28] and the regulations give additional flexibilities on income exclusions.[29]

---

[24] 42 U.S.C. 1786(d)(2).

[25] 42 U.S.C. 1786(d). 7 C.F.R. 246.7 also defines income and provides additional state options for income exclusion rules.

[26] 7 C.F.R. 246.2 defines family as "a group of related or nonrelated individuals who are living together as one economic unit, except that residents of a homeless facility or an institution shall not all be considered as members of a single family."

[27] 7 C.F.R. 246.7(d)(2)(i) provides states flexibility on the time frame of income counting, "In determining the income eligibility of an applicant, the State agency may instruct local agencies to consider the income of the family during the past 12 months and the family's current rate of income to determine which indicator more accurately reflects the family's status. However, persons from families with adult members who are unemployed shall be eligible based on income during the period of unemployment if the loss of income causes the current rate of income to be less than the State or local agency's income guidelines for Program eligibility."

[28] 42 U.S.C. 1786(d)(2)(B).

[29] See generally 7 C.F.R. 246.7(d)(2).

Table 3. WIC Income Eligibility Guidelines, 185% of Federal Poverty Level Effective from July 1, 2016, to June 30, 2017

Family/Household Size	48 States, District of Columbia, Territories	Alaska	Hawaii
1	$21,978	$27,454	$25,290
2	$29,637	$37,037	$34,096
3	$37,296	$46,620	$42,902
4	$44,955	$56,203	$51,708
5	$52,614	$65,786	$60,514
6	$60,273	$75,369	$69,320
7	$67,951	$84,952	$78,126
8	$75,647	$94,572	$86,969
Each additional family member	+$7,696	+$9,620	+$8,843

Source: USDA-FNS website, http://www.fns.usda.gov/wic/wic-income-eligibility-guidelines (also published in the *Federal Register*).

Note: Annual thresholds are provided here, but the state agency may determine income based on a shorter time frame.

The second pathway, adjunctive eligibility, deems an applicant income-eligible based on their participation in certain means-tested programs. Applicants that currently receive or are eligible to receive Supplemental Nutrition Assistance Program (SNAP), Medicaid, or Temporary Assistance for Needy Families (TANF) are adjunctively eligible.[30] Recent years' data—from a biennial USDA-FNS study using states' participant data—show that Medicaid has been consistently the most frequent source of adjunctive eligibility for WIC participants. Figure 2 displays the percentage of participants reporting participation in TANF, SNAP, and Medicaid. In April 2014, taking into account multiple program participation, 72.8% of WIC participants' income eligibility was

[30] 42 U.S.C. 1786(d)(2)(A). State agencies also have the option to deem applicants adjunctively eligible based on their participation in other state-administered programs as long as the programs have income eligibility guidelines at or below the state agency's WIC income guidelines and routinely require documentation of income (e.g., state-funded General Assistance programs). See 7 C.F.R. 246.7.

determined through adjunctive eligibility.[31] See Appendix Table A-2 for more detail on WIC participants' cross-program enrollment.

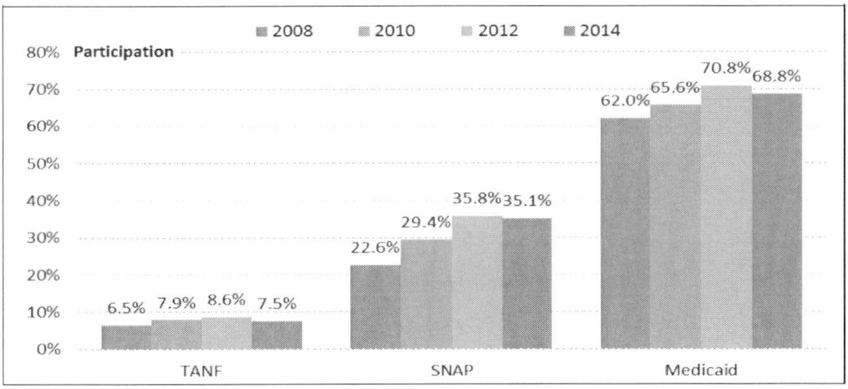

Source: CRS adaptation of B. Thorn, C. Tadler, and N. Huret et al., *WIC Participant and Program Characteristics 2014*, U.S. Department of Agriculture, Food and Nutrition Service, Final Report, Alexandria, VA, November, 2015, p. 33, Figure III.1.

Notes: The source of these data notes that these data likely underestimate participation in TANF, SNAP, and Medicaid. Reasons for underreporting include (1) information is recorded at time of certification and some participants are referred to these programs after certification, and (2) variations in office information systems and documentation policies.

Figure 2. Participants Reporting Participation in TANF, SNAP, Medicaid; 2008, 2010, 2012, 2014.

Because some states have income eligibility thresholds for SNAP and Medicaid that are above 185% of the federal poverty level, it is possible for WIC participants to have incomes over 185% of the federal poverty level. According to 2014 report data, 1.6% of WIC participants reported income above 185%.[32] The vast majority of participants reporting income (74.1%) are at or below the federal poverty level.[33]

---

[31] B. Thorn, C. Tadler, and N.Huret et al., *WIC Participant and Program Characteristics 2014*, U.S. Department of Agriculture, Food and Nutrition Service, Final Report, Alexandria, VA, November, 2015, p. 33. (Hereinafter cited as *WIC Participant and Program Characteristics 2014.*)

[32] Ibid. at p. 44.

[33] Ibid. Over 9% of participant data includes missing or ambiguous income data.

Nutritional Risk

Applicants must be at nutritional risk to qualify for WIC benefits, a rule that is unique to the WIC program, compared to other food assistance programs. Federal law recognizes five major types of nutritional risk,[34] falling into two broad categories: "medically based risks" and "diet-based risks."[35] Medically based risks include health conditions such as anemia, underweight, maternal age, history of pregnancy complications, or poor pregnancy outcomes. Diet-based risks refer to conditions that predispose applicants to inadequate nutritional patterns such as homelessness and migrancy.

To determine nutritional risk, a "competent professional authority," such as a physician, nutritionist, or nurse, must conduct a medical and/or nutritional assessment that includes the collection of anthropometric and biochemical measures, medical history, and dietary information from applicants and participants.[36] This assessment allows WIC providers to tailor participant benefits and services.[37]

Residential Eligibility and Immigration Status

Applicants must reside within the state in which their eligibility is determined and cannot participate in WIC at more than one WIC clinic at

---

[34] 42 U.S.C. 1786(a)(8). *Nutritional risk* is defined as "(A) detrimental or abnormal nutritional conditions detectable by biochemical or anthropometric measurements; (B) other documented nutritionally related medical conditions; (C) dietary deficiencies that impair or endanger health; (D) conditions that directly affect the nutritional health of a person, including alcoholism or drug abuse; or (E) conditions that predispose persons to inadequate nutritional patterns or nutritionally related medical conditions, including, but not limited to, homelessness and migrancy."

[35] See USDA-FNS website, "Frequently Asked Questions about WIC," http://www.fns.usda.gov/wic/frequently-asked- questions-about-wic#2.

[36] Per WIC law, " 'Competent professional authority' means physicians, nutritionists, registered nurses, dietitians, or State or local medically trained health officials, or persons designated by physicians or State or local medically trained health officials, in accordance with standards prescribed by the Secretary, as being competent professionally to evaluate nutritional risk." Section 17 (b)(3) of the Child Nutrition Act of 1966 (codified at 42 U.S.C. 1786(b)(3)).

[37] Oliveira and Frazão, EIB-134 (2015), p.5.; 42 U.S.C. 1786(f)(12), 7 C.F.R. 17(f)(12).

the same time. WIC state agencies have the option to limit WIC participation to U.S. citizens, nationals, and qualified aliens.[38]

Other Eligibility Issues

Certification Period

Once certified eligible for WIC, participants are eligible for a certain period of time. At the end of a certification period, eligible participants must be recertified to continue receiving benefits. At recertification, the WIC clinic will confirm that the participant is still eligible for benefits (including nutritional risk) and may adjust benefits if categorical status and/or nutritional needs change. The lengths of WIC certification periods vary by participant category, but in general, participants are eligible to receive benefits for a six-month period. Pregnant women are certified for the duration of their pregnancy and up to six weeks postpartum. Breastfeeding women are certified for six-month periods up to one year after delivery, while non-breastfeeding women are certified only up to six months after delivery. States have options to certify infants through their first birthday and/or children for up to one-year periods.[39]

Priority System and Waiting Lists

Federal regulations require states to use a priority system to manage WIC applicant waiting lists, in the event that limited funding prevents all eligible applicants from being served. Because WIC funding is discretionary, the number of participants served by the program is limited by the level of funding appropriated by Congress (and the allocation of these funds by USDA-FNS to each state). However, since the late 1990s funding provided has been adequate to serve all eligible applicants.[40] As a result, the priority system has largely gone unused in recent years—though

[38] 7 C.F.R. 246.7(c)(3).
[39] 42 U.S.C. 1786(d)(3).
[40] Oliveira and Frazão, EIB-134 (2015), p.19.

the issue of WIC waiting lists is often brought up by program advocates in budget-related debates.[41]

In the event that limited funding prevents all eligible applicants from participating in the program, local agencies are to create and maintain a waiting list of applicants seeking benefits.[42] Using a seven-point priority system, applicants are prioritized on the waiting list to ensure that those with the greatest nutritional risk and overall need can receive benefits.[43] Typically, applicants with medically based nutritional risks (e.g., anemia) are prioritized over those with only diet-based nutritional risks (e.g., conditions that may lead to inadequate diet). Additionally, certain participant categories—infants, pregnant women, and breastfeeding women—are given higher priority levels than other categories such as children and non-breastfeeding women.

BENEFITS AND SERVICES PROVIDED

The WIC program provides grants to states to provide benefits redeemable for specified supplemental foods (i.e., the WIC food package) and specified services. In addition to foods, WIC participants receive nutrition education, breastfeeding promotion and support, and referrals to healthcare and social services. Recent WIC grants to states for food costs as well as Nutrition Services and Administration (NSA) are displayed in Table 2, with historical funding in Table A1.

Supplemental Food Package

Typically, WIC participants receive vouchers/checks or an electronic benefit transfer (EBT) card, which are then redeemed for specific

---

[41] See, for example, Douglas A. Greenaway, National WIC Association, October 2013 blog post, https://www.nwica.org/blog/what-congress-can-do-to-keep-wic-doors-open-for-mothers-and-youngchildren#.VVT1X5PAOEI.

[42] 7 C.F.R. 246.7(f)(1).

[43] 7 C.F.R. 246.7(e)(4).

supplemental foods, and in some respects tailored to the specific participant's needs. The federal food package regulations and the basis for states' approved food lists are discussed in this section. More information about the delivery of benefits and states' food lists is provided in a subsequent section, "Redemption of Food Benefits and Related Cost Containment Policies."

Federal Requirements for WIC-Eligible Foods

The supplemental food package in a given state is the result of federal regulation and state policies.[44] Federal regulations list seven food packages, including eligible foods and their quantities, based on participant characteristics such as pregnancy status, breastfeeding practices, the age of children or infants, and dietary needs. Food items within the seven food packages include milk, juice, cereal, eggs, whole-wheat bread, legumes and peanut butter, cheese, canned fish, infant formula, infant cereal, and infant fruits, vegetables, and meats.[45] State agencies create their eligible food lists within this framework.[46] For instance, two states may make different brands of infant cereals WIC-eligible but both states' choices will meet the federal regulatory cereal requirements for sugar and fiber.[47] States' WIC food selections are a prime way that states can control costs and make their WIC grants go further.

---

[44] "Supplemental foods" is defined in federal WIC law as "those foods containing nutrients determined by nutritional research to be lacking in the diets of pregnant, breastfeeding, and postpartum women, infants, and children and foods that promote the health of the population served by the program authorized by this section [WIC], as indicated by relevant nutrition science, public health concerns, and cultural eating patterns, as prescribed by the Secretary [of Agriculture]. State agencies may, with the approval of the Secretary, substitute different foods providing the nutritional equivalent of foods prescribed by the Secretary, to allow for different cultural eating patterns." 42 U.S.C. 1786(b)(14).

[45] 7 C.F.R. 246.10(e). See Table 4 for the minimum requirements, specifications, and substitutions permitted for supplemental foods. WIC approved food lists vary considerably by state. A list of each state agency's WIC approved food list can be found on USDA-FNS's website: http://www.fns.usda.gov/wic/links-state-agency-wic-approved-foodlists.

[46] 7 C.F.R. 246.10(e).

[47] See state agency websites for state-specific WIC food lists. List of state agency websites available at http://www.fns.usda.gov/wic-state-agency-contacts.

The bulk of participants' benefits are for specific foods, but certain participants also receive a cash value voucher (CVV) for a specified monthly dollar amount to be redeemed for fruits and vegetables.[48] Figure 3 summarizes the federal WIC food packages—noting which packages include a CVV.

WIC law, as amended in 2004 and 2010, requires USDA to conduct periodic ("not less than every 10 years") scientific reviews of foods included in the WIC food packages and to change the regulations as necessary.[49] The current federal food package regulations, discussed in this section and displayed in Figure 3, are largely the result of significant revisions that began in 2003 with meetings of the National Academy of Sciences' Institute of Medicine (IOM) and continued with a 2007 interim rule that was finalized in 2014, with an added change (allowing CVV purchases of white potatoes) from Congress through the FY2015 appropriations law. The 2003 revision had been the first major revision since the 1970s. Note: In 2016, the IOM was renamed the Health and Medicine Division (HMD) of the National Academies of Sciences, Engineering, and Medicine (NASEM).[50]

Since the 2014 final rule, USDA-FNS engaged IOM/HMD for further review and assessment of the WIC food package studies. HMD convened an expert committee, and has since produced three reports, the third and final of which is expected to form the basis for FNS's next revision of the WIC food packages.[51]

---

[48] See Table 4 of paragraph 7 C.F.R. 246.10 (e)(12) for cash value voucher limitations.

[49] 42 U.S.C. 1786(h)(11)(C). Periodic reviews added by Child Nutrition and WIC Reauthorization Act of 2004 (P.L. 108-265); 10-year timeframe added by Healthy, Hunger-Free Kids Act of 2010 (P.L. 111-296).

[50] In March 2016, IOM was renamed the Health and Medicine Division (HMD) of the National Academies of Sciences, Engineering and Medicine.

[51] The HMD committee produced three reports: (1) Review of WIC Food Packages: An Evaluation of White Potatoes in the Cash Value Voucher (February 3, 2015); (2) Review of WIC Food Packages: Proposed Framework for Revisions: Interim Report (November 30, 2015); (3) Review of WIC Food Packages: Improving Balance and Choice (January 5, 2017). See http://nationalacademies.org/hmd/Reports/2017/review-of-wic-food-packages-improvingbalance-and-choice.aspx.

Package #	Participant Category	Age/Duration	Foods	Cash Value Voucher Amount[1]
I	Infants[2]	Ages 0 through 5 months old	Infant formula	-
II	Infants[2]	Ages 6 through 11 months old	Infant formula, infant cereal, infant fruits and vegetables, infant meat	-
III	Participants with qualifying conditions (includes women, infants, children)[3]	Same as participant's category	With medical documentation: infant formula, exempt infant formula, or WIC-eligible medical foods, plus all of the foods in the packages to which they would have been eligible in the absence of their special medical needs	Same as participant's category
IV	Children	Ages 1 through 4 years old	Juice, milk, breakfast cereal, eggs, whole-wheat bread, legumes or peanut butter, fruits and vegetables	$8
V	Pregnant and Partially Breastfeeding Women	Pregnant women: until mother gives birth; Partially breastfeeding women: up to 1 year after giving birth	Juice, milk, breakfast cereal, eggs, whole-wheat bread, legumes and peanut butter, fruits and vegetables	$10
VI	Postpartum Women (non-breastfeeding)	Up to 6 months postpartum	Juice, milk, breakfast cereal, eggs, legumes or peanut butter, fruits and vegetables	$10
VII	Fully Breastfeeding Women	Up to 1 year	Juice, milk, cheese, breakfast cereal, eggs, whole-wheat bread, legumes and peanut butter, canned fish, fruits and vegetables	$10

Source: CRS adaptation of Victor Oliveira and Elizabeth Frazão, *The WIC Program: Background, Trends, and Economic Issues, 2015 Edition*, EIB-134, U.S. Department of Agriculture, Economic Research Service, January 2015, p. 7, Table 2.

Notes: In addition to the foods listed here, the federal food package regulations give states certain substitution options such as yogurt as a substitute for milk for Food Packages III-IV.

(1) Provided per month. Cash value voucher amounts are adjusted for inflation according to rules in 7 C.F.R. 246.16;

(2) Three infant feeding options are available under these packages, depending whether the infant is fully, partially, or not breastfeeding;

(3) For any participant with a "documented qualifying condition," substitutions to the conventional foods may be made.

Figure 3. Overview of the Seven WIC Food Packages; Details at 7 C.F.R. 246.10.

Appendix B provides further detail on the WIC food package updates and proposed food package updates discussed in this section.

Issuance of Food Benefits

At a WIC clinic (local agency), a "competent professional authority" will assign an applicant to one of seven food packages (Figure 3). Participants are eligible to receive up to the maximum food benefits as determined by medical and nutritional need, not household income. Prescribed foods are typically reassessed at each recertification or when a participant's status changes (e.g., after a pregnant participant gives birth). Food package benefits are usually issued monthly.[52]

Currently, all but two state agencies have participants redeem their benefits at authorized WIC vendors (retailers).[53] Most are issuing benefits through paper checks/vouchers, but (as of March 2017) 24 state agencies have implemented an electronic benefit transfer (EBT) system statewide.[54] These benefit redemption concepts are discussed further in "Retail Food Delivery Systems and the Transition to EBT."

Nutrition Education, Breastfeeding, and Referral Services

In addition to food benefits, WIC also provides nutrition education and related support. States are required to ensure that nutrition education, including breastfeeding promotion and drug abuse education, is available to all pregnant, postpartum, and breastfeeding participants in the program.[55] States develop and coordinate nutrition education services and oversee and support the administration of these benefits at local agencies. Under federal guidelines, WIC nutrition education must emphasize the relationship between nutrition, physical activity, and health and it must assist each participant in improving health status and achieving a positive change in dietary and physical activity habits.[56] Nutrition education is provided through a number of approaches, including individual consultations, group counseling sessions, and online educational modules.

---

[52] Participants can be issued up to a three-month supply of food benefits vouchers at a time with each voucher typically valid for a 30-day period. 7 C.F.R. 246.12 (r)(5).

[53] WIC state agencies may choose from three types of food delivery systems: retail, home delivery, and/or direct distribution. Currently, all state agencies except Vermont and Mississippi operate retail food delivery systems. Vermont operates a home delivery system and Mississippi operates a direct distribution delivery system in which participants pick up food from designated facilities operated by the state agency. Both agencies are scheduled to switch to the retail food delivery system as part of their transition to EBT.

[54] USDA-FNS, http://www.fns.usda.gov/wic/wic-ebt-activities.

[55] 42 U.S.C. 1786(e).

[56] See 7 C.F.R. 246.11(b).

Though WIC does provide infant formula for infants whose mothers do not breastfeed, or do not exclusively breastfeed, WIC also promotes and supports breastfeeding in a variety of ways. States must establish standards and practices for breastfeeding promotion within nutrition education services.[57] Additionally, states must spend an annual average of at least $21 per pregnant and breastfeeding woman to promote breastfeeding.[58] Examples of breastfeeding promotion and support services include breastfeeding peer counselors, lactation consultants, classes and support groups, educational materials, and a breastfeeding hotline for questions.[59] According to USDA-FNS, breastfeeding initiation has increased in recent years. 69.8% of WIC infants 6 to 13 months old were breastfed at some point in 2014, an increase from 67.1% in 2012.[60]

In an effort to integrate available services, state and local WIC agencies often provide applicants and participants with information on other health-related and public assistance programs (such as Medicaid, SNAP, and immunizations).[61] WIC law requires that states provide Medicaid information to individuals that are income-eligible and not participating.[62]

---

[57] 7 C.F.R. 246.11(c)(7). See USDA's WIC Works Resource System for nutrition education materials used by states, http://wicworks.nal.usda.gov/nutrition-education.

[58] 42 U.S.C. 1786(h)(3)(E).

[59] For further information on WIC's provision of breastfeeding and support services, see related USDA-FNS resources available at http://www.fns.usda.gov/wic/breastfeeding-promotion-and-support-wic.

[60] Breastfeeding initiation refers to the incidence of breastfeeding rather than the duration of breastfeeding, meaning an infant was fed breast milk at least once or more. See, *WIC Participant and Program Characteristics 2014,* pp. 141-147. Table VI.2. (on p. 145) indicates the rate of breastfeeding initiation has been increasing since 1998, although there are limitations to comparing the data across years.

[61] WIC regulations require states to make such referrals, 7 C.F.R. 246.7(b).

[62] 42 U.S.C. 1786(e)(4): "The State agency ... shall provide to individuals applying for the program under this section, or reapplying at the end of their certification period, written information about the Medicaid program and referral to such program or to agencies authorized to determine presumptive eligibility for such program, if such individuals are not participating in such program and appear to have family income below the applicable maximum income limits for such program."

REDEMPTION OF FOOD BENEFITS AND RELATED COST CONTAINMENT POLICIES

State agencies, under federal guidelines, design and oversee the delivery of food benefits to participants. As stated earlier, almost all state agencies currently provide benefits using a voucher or EBT card for redemption at an authorized vendor. This section provides an overview of benefit redemption, states' transitions to EBT, authorization and management of vendors, and related cost containment policies.

Retail Food Delivery Systems and the Transition to EBT

Currently, most states have their participants redeem WIC benefits using a paper food instrument in the form of a check or voucher that specifies the types and quantities of foods that can be purchased at an authorized WIC vendor. Vendors send vouchers to the states, and the states reimburse vendors (using food grant funds) for WIC benefit redemptions. With paper vouchers, each will typically be redeemable for a group of approved foods (e.g., milk and eggs for the month), and WIC participants will have to redeem the entire group in the same transaction or lose the benefits if they make a partial transaction (e.g., only milk with the "milk and eggs" voucher).

WIC's 2010 reauthorization included the requirement that state agencies transition to using electronic benefit transfer (EBT) by October 1, 2020 (the end of FY2020).[63] SNAP underwent the transition from paper food stamps to EBT from 1988 to 2004.[64] WIC EBT (referred to by some states and stakeholders as "eWIC") replaces vouchers with a card, similar to a debit card, which keeps track of remaining and redeemed benefits.

[63] 42 U.S.C. 1786(h)(12) as amended by Healthy, Hunger-Free Kids Act of 2010 (P.L. 111-296).

[64] See USDA-FNS website "A Short History of SNAP," http://www.fns.usda.gov/snap/short-history-snap.

Policy rationales for this transition include program integrity considerations as well as improved services for participants and vendors.[65]

EBT, for instance, allows food benefits to be redeemed for each item individually or in groupings of the participant's choice. The WIC technology is more complex than SNAP's, however, and state agencies are at varying stages of making the transition.[66] 24 state agencies (20 states and 4 Indian Tribal Organizations), as of March 2017, have fully transitioned to WIC EBT.[67] The fruit and vegetable cash-value voucher (CVV) is included in a transition to EBT, and so some states and stakeholders have begun referring to it instead as a cash-value *benefit* (CVB).

States' Cost Containment through Approved Foods

Approved Food Lists

Referred to earlier, the specific types and quantities of approved foods for redemption are a prime way states control food costs. In practice, states often control food costs by limiting participants' food-item selection to specific brands, economically priced package sizes and product forms, or least-cost brands. States' approved food lists, along with geographic variation in food costs, explain much of the variation between average food

---

[65] In the report accompanying the 2010 reauthorization, the Senate committee wrote, in part, "Updating technology in the WIC Program will allow State WIC staff at all levels to perform operations more effectively and efficiently, increasing accountability and streamlining program monitoring and business practices through electronic solutions. At the clinic level it will enhance client services by improving clinic efficiencies. EBT will improve access to prescribed WIC foods by allowing the participant to shop for benefits when they want to and in the amounts they wish to purchase. EBT will also simplify the retail point-of-sale transaction and will reduce participant stigma and improve the shopping experience. WIC benefit redemption and payment for WIC transactions will be vastly improved for retailers using EBT." S.Rept. 111-178, p. 10.

[66] For additional resources and guidance on the transition to WIC EBT, see USDA-FNS's webpage on WIC Electronic Benefits Transfer (EBT) Guidance and Resources: http://www.fns.usda.gov/wic/wic-electronic-benefits-transfer-ebtguidance. See also Diane Phillips, Loren Bell, and Ruth Morgan, et al., *Transition to EBT in WIC: Review of Impact and Examination of Participant Redemption Patterns*, Altarum Institute, Final Report, September 8, 2014, http://altarum.org/publications/transition-to-ebt-in-wic-review-of-impact-and-examination-of-participant-redemptionpatterns.

[67] See state agencies EBT implementation at USDA-FNS's WIC EBT Activity Map and Status Report, updated monthly, http://www.fns.usda.gov/wic/wic-ebt-activities.

package costs in states. In FY2015, the average monthly food package cost was over $43 nationwide; individual state agencies' average monthly food package costs ranged from around $29 to $96.[68] However, states balance cost containment considerations with participant satisfaction, as an approved food list that is too limited may stifle participation.[69]

Infant Formula (and Other Food) Rebates

Manufacturers' rebates for infant formula (and some other foods) also serve to contain WIC food costs.

Over time, one of the ways that WIC has controlled costs has been to require competitive bidding for infant formula, which has resulted in infant formula being available to states at well below market costs, especially due to manufacturers' discounts in the form of rebates to states. Infant formula has been shown to be the most expensive WIC food category. A study of FY2010 found that, without infant formula rebates, infant formula would have accounted for 42% of WIC food costs in FY2010; after rebates, formula costs were only 20%.[70]

Infant formula manufacturers submit bids through a state's (and, in some cases, alliances of states) competitive bidding process, and the contract is awarded to the manufacturer with the lowest price. The requirement that states pursue such cost containment systems for infant formula was added by the Child Nutrition and WIC Reauthorization Act of 1989 (P.L. 101-147), although some states had begun to enter into these arrangements prior to the law's passage and implementation.[71]

---

[68] U.S. Department of Agriculture, Food and Nutrition Service., *WIC Program, Annual State Level Data: FY 2009- 2014 - Average Monthly Food Cost Per Person*, June 5, 2015, http://www.fns.usda.gov/pd/wic-program.

[69] For more information on the assessment of WIC cost-containment practices, see John A. Kirlin and Nancy Cole, *Assessment of WIC Cost-Containment Practices*, USDA-ERS, Report Number 31, Washington, DC, May 2003, https://www.ers.usda.gov/webdocs/publications/fanrr31/35814_fanrr31.pdf?v=42499.

[70] Tracy Vericker, Chen Zhen, and Shawn Karns, *Fiscal Year 2010 WIC Food Cost Report*, USDA Food and Nutrition Service, August 2013, p. 16.

[71] See 42 U.S.C. 1786(h)(8). Provision creates certain exemptions from these cost containment requirements (e.g., Indian Tribal Organization agencies with less than 1,000 participants). Further history of infant formula rebates is provided in Steven Carlson, Robert Greenstein, and Zoë Neuberger, *WIC's Competitive Bidding Process for Infant Formula Is Highly Cost-Effective*, Center on Budget and Policy Priorities, June 24, 2015, pp. 2-4,

A rebate contract is a legal agreement between an infant formula manufacturer and a state (or multistate alliance).[72] In a rebate contract, the state agency receives a rebate payment from the manufacturer, with total rebate payments depending upon how much infant formula was ultimately purchased with WIC benefits.[73] The manufacturer receives the exclusive right to sell formula to the state's WIC participants.[74] (Note: Some states competitively bid their milk- and soy-based formulas separately, so WIC participants buy formula from two manufacturers rather than a sole source.) WIC-authorized retailers are reimbursed for the "full" retail price of the infant formula, but state agencies then submit their reimbursements to the manufacturers for rebates.

Though the rebate may impact the manufacturers' profit on the WIC purchases, economic research indicates that the manufacturer who wins the state's WIC business also gains non-WIC business in the state.[75]

Infant formula rebates have significantly defrayed the costs of operating the WIC program. USDA-ERS estimates that, in FY2013, rebates generated $1.9 billion in savings.[76] USDA-ERS also found that infant formula manufacturers in FY2013 were providing percentage

---

http://www.cbpp.org/research/food-assistance/wics-competitive-bidding-process-for-infant-formula-is-highly-cost.

[72] Over half of the WIC state agencies that operate a competitive rebate system do so as part of a multistate alliance. For a list of multistate alliance states, see Victor Oliveira, Elizabeth Frazão, and David Smallwood, *Trends in Infant Formula Rebate Contracts: Implications for the WIC Program*, USDA-ERS, EIB-119, December 2013, p. 7, https://www.ers.usda.gov/webdocs/publications/eib119/41312_eib119_summary.pdf.

[73] For more information on formula rebate contracts and program implications, see USDA-ERS's study: David E. Davis and Victor Oliveira, *Manufacturers' Bids for WIC Infant Formula Rebate, 2003-2013*, U.S. Department of Agriculture, Economic Research Service, Number 142, July 2015, https://www.ers.usda.gov/webdocs/publications/eib142/53266_eib142.pdf?v=42314.

[74] WIC does make exceptions to the contract brand for participants with religious or medical needs. 7 C.F.R. 246.10(d).

[75] Using retailer data from 30 states in 2004-2009, a USDA-ERS analysis found that when states switched brands the prior manufacturer's total sales severely dropped and the new manufacturer's sales increased; ERS found that the benefits of the contract "spill over" to non-WIC purchases. Victor Oliveira, "Winner Takes (Almost) All: How WIC Affects the Infant Formula Market," *Amber Waves*, September 1, 2011.

[76] David E. Davis and Victor Oliveira, *Manufacturers' Bids for WIC Infant Formula Rebate Contracts, 2003-2013*, USDA Economic Research Service, Number 142, July 2015, p. 2.

discounts ranging from 77% to 98%, with 21 state agencies receiving discounts of 95% or greater.[77]

Although the law does not require states to pursue competitive bidding for other foods, some states have pursued rebate contracts for infant foods. According to March 2017 USDA-FNS data, eight WIC state agencies had rebate contracts for infant foods.[78]

Vendor Authorization and Management[79]

WIC uses the term "vendors" to describe the retailers that states authorize to accept WIC benefits.[80] In FY2013, there were over 48,000 WIC authorized vendors nationwide.[81] The sections that follow provide an overview of how states authorize WIC vendors and federal and state price-related policy impacting cost containment in WIC.

States' Authorization of Vendors

Vendors include a variety of retailers from supermarkets to convenience stores to military commissaries. State agencies are responsible for setting criteria and authorizing WIC vendors, within the framework of federal law and regulations. State agencies select and authorize vendors based on a set of criteria, such as competitive pricing, minimum stocking

[77] Victor Oliveira, Elizabeth Frazão, and David Smallwood, *Trends in Infant Formula Rebate Contracts: Implications for the WIC Program*, USDA-ERS, EIB-119, December 2013, p. 9, https://www.ers.usda.gov/webdocs/publications/ eib119/41313_eib119.pdf?v=41645.

[78] Data provided by USDA-FNS staff. The eight states are New York, Ohio, Texas, and one multi-state alliance (Connecticut, Maine, Massachusetts, New Hampshire, and Rhode Island).

[79] Further detail about these policies is provided in S. Gleason, R. Morgan, and L. Bell, et al., *2013 WIC Vendor Management Study*, USDA-FNS, Final Report, Alexandria, VA, November 2013, pp. 2-5, http://www.fns.usda.gov/ sites/default/files/2013WICVendor.pdf.

[80] 7 C.F.R. 246.2, in part: "*Vendor* means a sole proprietorship, partnership, cooperative association, corporation, or other business entity operating one or more stores authorized by the State agency to provide authorized supplemental foods to participants under a retail food delivery system."

[81] S. Gleason, R. Morgan, and L. Bell, et al., *2013 WIC Vendor Management Study*, USDA-FNS, Final Report, Alexandria, VA, November 2013, p. 1, http://www.fns.usda.gov/ sites/default/files/2013WICVendor.pdf.

requirements of supplemental foods, and business integrity.[82] If a vendor satisfies the state's criteria and participates in the agency's WIC training, it may enter into a vendor agreement with the state agency, thereby agreeing to comply with the state's rules and regulations.

Overseeing Vendors

As discussed earlier, WIC food benefits are provided in the form of specific foods, rather than a dollar amount of benefits (the cash value voucher/benefit is the exception). This can set up challenges for program spending, as participants are less sensitive to the price of goods and vendors can potentially take advantage of this. Therefore, states consider and monitor WIC vendors' pricing as a means of cost containment. For instance, federal law requires (1) the establishment of vendor "peer groups" and (2) additional strictures for vendors that receive over 50% of their revenue from WIC transactions. These policies, discussed further below, were added to WIC law in the 2004 reauthorization.[83]

Federal law requires states to establish a vendor peer group system for their WIC vendors. State agencies group vendors based on shared characteristics or criteria that affect food prices and compare prices within the group. Groups are based upon factors such as store size, geographic location, sales, and/or type of ownership. For example, large chain groceries may be grouped together as one peer group, while pharmacies may be grouped in another. States establish competitive price criteria for each peer group, with most states establishing a Maximum Allowable Reimbursement Level (MARL) or the total maximum reimbursement rate for each WIC transaction.[84] When a vendor sends in a WIC voucher for reimbursement, the vendor will not be reimbursed above the MARL.

---

[82] Per federal regulation, states must set their own minimum stocking requirements but they must include at least two varieties of fruits, two varieties of vegetables, and one whole grain cereal. These and other federal requirements for states' vendor authorization are at 7 C.F.R. 246.12(g).

[83] 42 U.S.C. 1786(h)(11) (as amended by the Child Nutrition and WIC Reauthorization Act of 2004, P.L. 108-265). S.Rept. 108-279, pp. 53-57.

[84] 42 U.S.C. 1786(h)(11)(C),(E). Some states use the term MAR (Maximum Allowable Reimbursement).

Also per the 2004 reauthorization law, states enforce additional requirements for vendors that receive over half their revenue from WIC transactions. These stores have been colloquially referred to as "WIC-only" vendors and in WIC regulations are called "above-50-percent" (A50) vendors. The 2004 law restricted A50 stores from providing incentives or other free merchandise to customers, and states are also required to limit A50 maximum reimbursements to the average of all other stores in the state.[85] Not all states have A50 stores.[86]

At times, USDA and/or state agencies have imposed a vendor moratorium in states that have had issues managing cost containment and maintaining the integrity of existing WIC vendors. Under a vendor moratorium, no new vendors are authorized.[87]

CONCLUSION

Several aspects of the WIC program discussed in this primer—funding, eligible foods, and retail transactions—have been of interest to policymakers in the past and may continue to be in the future. Although the program has been reauthorized roughly every five years, interest in or debate over the program also arises in the context of annual appropriations deliberations. In light of budget laws' discretionary spending limits, congressional appropriators consider forecasted WIC need against other priorities. In addition to funding matters, moving forward, policymakers may be interested in overseeing the next update to the WIC food package regulations and states' transitions to EBT.

---

[85] See also 7 C.F.R. 246.12(g).

[86] According to administrative data provided by USDA-FNS, as of September 30, 2014, A50 vendors are authorized in 13 state agencies. The 13 state agencies are Arizona; California; Connecticut; Florida; Georgia; Louisiana; New Mexico; New York; Oklahoma; Puerto Rico; Texas; Wisconsin; and Wichita, Caddo, and Delaware Tribes. Nearly 80% of these stores are authorized in California and Puerto Rico.

[87] Recent examples of vendor moratoria include California (lifted effective February 1, 2015) and Louisiana (ongoing as of the date of this chapter). See California's "Notice of Final Moratorium Lift" http://www.cdph.ca.gov/programs/ wicworks/Documents/VendorAlerts/ WIC-Vendor-Alert-2015-01.pdf; Louisiana's vendor notice http://dhh.louisiana.gov/assets/ oph/nutrition/WIC/alerts/VendorAlerts2014/ VendorNotice_FederalMoratorium52214.pdf.

Along with the sources cited throughout the report, please see the text box below for a listing of additional resources which provide finer detail than was included in this overview.

Additional WIC Resources

- USDA-FNS WIC Website: http://www.fns.usda.gov/wic/women-infants-and-children-wic. Includes program descriptions, press releases, current policy guidance and regulations, and participation and spending data.
- USDA-FNS WIC Studies Website: http://www.fns.usda.gov/ops/wic-studies. Includes reports and studies on the WIC program such as
    - WIC Participant and Program Characteristics 2014: https://www.fns.usda.gov/wic-participant-and-programcharacteristics-2014. Report summarizes the demographic characteristics of WIC participants nationwide in April 2014.
    - 2013 WIC Vendor Management Study: http://www.fns.usda.gov/2013-wic-vendor-management-study. Study estimates the level of vendor errors in WIC by examining compliance buys using paper- or EBT-based food instruments.
    - National and State-level Estimates of WIC Eligibles and Program Reach, 2013: https://www.fns.usda.gov/nationaland-state-level-estimates-special-supplemental-nutrition-program-women-infants-and-childr-2. Report updates estimates on the number of people eligible for WIC benefits in 2013.
- FY2017 President's Budget Justification for USDA-FNS (pp. 32-74 to 32-90): http://www.obpa.usda.gov/32fns2017notes.pdf. Includes funding and program data, performance and evaluation data, along with general information on the WIC program.
- USDA-ERS Report: The WIC Program: Background, Trends, and Economic Issues, 2015 Edition: http://www.obpa.usda.gov/32fns2016notes.pdf. Report provides an overview of the WIC program, as well information on program trends and economic issues.
- WIC State Agency Contacts and Websites: http://www.fns.usda.gov/wic/wic-contacts. USDA-FNS maintains this list of state agencies' contact information and websites.

APPENDIX A. ADDITIONAL WIC DATA

Table A-1. WIC Participation and Costs FY1989-FY2016 Cost data in current dollars

Fiscal Year	Total Participation[b] (in thousands)	Federal Spending (in millions of dollars)[a]			Per Participant Monthly Food Cost
		Food Costs	Nutrition Services and Administration (NSA) Costs	Total (including other costs)[c]	
1989	4,119	$1,489.4	$416.5	$1,908.9	$30.13
1990	4,517	1,636.8	478.7	2,120.4	30.20
1991	4,893	1,751.9	544.0	2,298.3	29.84
1992	5,403	1,960.5	632.7	2,598.2	30.24
1993	5,921	2,115.1	705.6	2,825.5	29.77
1994	6,477	2,325.2	834.4	3,164.4	29.92
1995	6,894	2,511.6	904.6	3,429.7	30.36
1996	7,186	2,689.9	985.1	3,688.5	31.19
1997	7,407	2,815.5	1,008.2	3,837.2	31.68
1998	7,367	2,808.1	1,061.4	3,880.0	31.76
1999	7,311	2,851.6	1,063.9	3,926.0	32.50
2000	7,192	2,853.1	1,102.6	3,966.1	33.06
2001	7,306	3,007.9	1,110.6	4,132.6	34.31
2002	7,491	3,129.7	1,182.3	4,322.7	34.82
2003	7,631	3,230.3	1,260.0	4,504.7	35.28
2004	7,904	3,562.0	1,272.4	4,865.7	37.55
2005	8,023	3,602.8	1,335.5	4,968.4	37.42
2006	8,088	3,597.5	1,402.6	5,050.6	37.07
2007	8,285	3,881.1	1,479.0	5,389.1	39.04
2008	8,705	4,534.0	1,607.6	6,169.3	43.40
2009	9,122	4,640.9	1,788.0	6,451.9	42.40
2010	9,175	4,561.8	1,907.9	6,671.3	41.43
2011	8,961	5,020.2	1,961.3	7,159.6	46.69
2012	8,908	4,809.9	1,877.8	6,782.9	45.00
2013	8,663	4,497.1	1,881.6	6,463.1	43.26
2014	8,258	4,325.7	1,903.3	6,277.5	43.65
2015	8,024	4,176	1,922	6,210	43.37
2016	7,696	3,949	1,948	5,960	42.76

Source: USDA-FNS data, as of March 8, 2017.

[a] USDA-FNS describes these data as both outlays and unliquidated obligations for the given year.

[b] Average monthly participation in the given year.

[c] This total includes Food and NSA as well as EBT, Infrastructure, Breastfeeding Peer Counselors, and other federal WIC costs.

Table A-2. Number and Percentage of WIC Participants Reporting Participation in Other Programs Participant reports at certification

By Programs		
Program	Number of Participants	% of U.S. WIC Participation[a]
TANF	699,952	7.5%
SNAP	3,268,231	35.8%
Medicaid	6,402,851	68.8%
TANF, SNAP, and/or Medicaid	6.769,683	72.8%
By Combination of Programs, Where Applicable		
Program	Number of Participants	% of U.S. WIC Participation
TANF, SNAP, and Medicaid	557,853	6.0%
TANF and SNAP	29,099	0.3%
TANF and Medicaid	61,692	0.7%
SNAP and Medicaid	2,394,853	25.7%
TANF only	51,308	0.6%
	286,426	3.1%
Medicaid only	3,388,453	36.4%
Do not participate in TANF, SNAP, or Medicaid	1,960,470	21.1%
Not reported	573,100	6.2%
Total WIC Participation	9,303,253	100.0%

Source: B. Thorn, C. Tadler, and N.Huret et al., *WIC Participant and Program Characteristics 2014*, U.S. Department of Agriculture, Food and Nutrition Service, Final Report, Alexandria, VA, November, 2015, p. 34, Table III.1.

Notes: Source notes that this data likely underestimates participation in TANF, SNAP, and Medicaid. Reasons for underreporting include (1) information is recorded at time of certification and some participants are referred to these programs after certification, and (2) variations in office information systems and documentation policies.

[a.] Total of this column exceeds 100% because of participation in combinations of programs.

APPENDIX B. REVISIONS OF WIC FOOD PACKAGES, 2003-PRESENT

2009 Changes to the WIC Food Packages

Effective October 1, 2009, USDA significantly revised the WIC food packages. These changes were made to reflect updates and revisions in nutrition science, public health concerns, and cultural eating patterns. The revised packages provide participants with a wider variety of foods, including whole grains, fruits, and vegetables; increase incentives for breastfeeding; and allow states greater flexibility in accommodating cultural preferences of participants. Before USDA embarked on this process to update the food packages, there had not been a major revision since the 1970s.[88]

In 2003, USDA-FNS contracted with the Institute of Medicine (IOM) to independently review the WIC food packages, in order to align them more closely with updated nutrition science.[89] IOM released its final report in 2005, recommending significant, though cost-neutral, changes to the food packages.[90] IOM's major recommendations included the addition of whole-wheat bread and infant foods including fruits, vegetables, and meats; revised food quantities and food package categories; additional foods for breastfeeding women and breastfed infants; providing new optional food-substitutions (such as soy milk and tofu); and the introduction of a cash-value voucher (CVV) redeemable for a specified dollar amount of fruits and vegetables.

In December 2007, USDA-FNS published an interim final rule to update the WIC food packages. This interim rule largely included the IOM's recommendations, and state agencies were required to implement the changes in their state lists by October 1, 2009.[91] While the interim final rule was in effect, USDA-FNS collected comments on its implementation,

---

[88] http://www.iom.edu/Reports/2005/WIC-Food-Packages-Time-for-a-Change/Actions-Taken.aspx.

[89] See USDA-FNS's Background: Revisions to the WIC Food Package for more information: http://www.fns.usda.gov/ wic/background-revisions-wic-food-package.

[90] National Research Council, *WIC Food Packages: Time for a Change* (Washington, DC: The National Academies Press, 2005).

[91] Department of Agriculture, Food and Nutrition Service, "Special Supplemental Nutrition Program for Women, Infants and Children (WIC): Revisions in the WIC Food Packages," 72 *Federal Register*, December 6, 2007. Under the Administrative Procedure Act (5 U.S.C. §553), if an agency has "good cause," it may issue a rule that becomes effective immediately and hold a comment period after the rule has already become effective. If the agency is persuaded by any of the comments received during that comment period and so chooses, it can later amend the rule in light of those comments.

receiving over 7,500 letters. The agency published a final rule in March 2014.[92]

About the White Potato Policy Changes[93]

The description of the WIC food packages in the "Supplemental Food Package" section of this chapter largely reflects the March 2014 final rule. Both the interim and final rules restricted the purchase of white potatoes, but a 2015 legislative change now allows their purchase.

One of the changes in the updated food packages was the inclusion of the CVV. Based on the 2005 IOM recommendations, these interim and final regulations did not allow participants to purchase white potatoes with the CVV. IOM cited the 2005 Dietary Guidelines for Americans for starchy vegetable consumption as well as food intake data showing that white potatoes, unlike many other vegetables, were already widely consumed.

This policy proved to be controversial in Congress and related proposals were included in the 112th and 113th Congress.[94] In December 2014, Congress enacted a FY2015 appropriations law that included a policy rider (Section 753 of P.L. 113-235) to change WIC's exclusion of white potatoes. The law barred USDA from excluding any vegetable (without added sugar, salt, or fat) from the WIC food packages, therefore

---

[92] Department of Agriculture, Food and Nutrition Service, "Special Supplemental Nutrition Program for Women, Infants and Children (WIC): Revisions in the WIC Food Packages," 79 *Federal Register* 12274 et seq., March 4, 2014. See also related USDA-FNS resources at http://www.fns.usda.gov/wic/final-rule-revisions-wic-food-packages.

[93] For further details on congressional and IOM actions around white potatoes in the food package, see CRS Insight IN10226, *WIC and White Potatoes: Understanding Recent News from the Institute of Medicine (IOM)*, by Randy Alison Aussenberg (available upon request).

[94] In the 113th Congress, a study of potatoes was ultimately proposed but not included in the 2014 farm bill (CRS Report R43332, *SNAP and Related Nutrition Provisions of the 2014 Farm Bill (P.L. 113-79)*); and the House Appropriations Committee's FY2014 bill included a policy rider that would have required inclusion of white potatoes, but the enacted law only included less powerful language in its Joint Explanatory Statement (CRS Report R43110, *Agriculture and Related Agencies: FY2014 and FY2013 (Post-Sequestration) Appropriations*).

allowing white potatoes. The provision also required USDA to conduct another review of the WIC food packages, and, based on the results of that review, white potatoes (or other vegetables) would either continue to be included or would return to being excluded. In response to the appropriations law, on December 30, 2014, FNS issued policy guidance to states for implementing the inclusion of white potatoes.[95] States were required to submit implementation plans to FNS by January 30, 2015. FNS's memo states that "state agencies are expected to complete all implementation actions as soon as possible, but no later than July 1, 2015."

IOM/HMD's WIC Food Package Review: 2015-Present

Note: In 2016, the IOM was renamed the Health and Medicine Division (HMD) of the National Academies of Sciences, Engineering, and Medicine (NASEM).[96]

Since the 2014 final rule, USDA-FNS engaged HMD for further review and assessment of the WIC food package studies. HMD convened an expert committee and has since produced three reports, the third and final of which is expected to form the basis for FNS's next revision of the WIC food packages.[97]

The first, published in February 2015, was a "letter report" regarding the inclusion of the white potatoes issue (this was the review required by P.L. 113-235). The committee evaluated the 2009 regulation and, along with recommendations on data collection and study topics, recommended that USDA allow white potatoes as a WIC-eligible vegetable for purchase

---

[95] http://www.fns.usda.gov/eligibility-white-potatoes-purchase-cash-value-voucher.

[96] See "Our Web Address & Division Name," http://www.nationalacademies.org/hmd/About-HMD/DivisionName.aspx.

[97] The HMD committee produced three reports: (1) *Review of WIC Food Packages: An Evaluation of White Potatoes in the Cash Value Voucher* (February 3, 2015); (2) *Review of WIC Food Packages: Proposed Framework for Revisions: Interim Report* (November 30, 2015); (3) *Review of WIC Food Packages: Improving Balance and Choice* (January 5, 2017). See http://nationalacademies.org/hmd/Activities/Nutrition/ReviewWICFoodPackages.aspx.

with the cash value voucher so long as this was consistent with the (forthcoming at that time) 2015 Dietary Guidelines for Americans.[98]

The second, published in November 2015, established a framework by which the HMD committee would subsequently evaluate the current WIC food packages and make findings in the final report.[99]

The third and final report of the series was published in January 2017; it is the HMD committee's final analysis of the current WIC food packages and includes recommendations for changes.[100] In general, the committee recommends increasing the amounts of the cash value voucher, servings of whole grains, and seafood, while decreasing juice, milk, legumes, peanut butter, infant vegetables, fruits, and meats. For all food packages for women and children, the committee recommends

- increasing the dollar amount of cash value vouchers;
- adding fish;
- increasing the amount of whole grains from 16 ounces to 24 ounces; and
- reducing the amounts of juice, dairy, legumes, and peanut butter.

HMD also recommended policy changes to encourage partial breastfeeding over the exclusively formula-feeding package. Additional recommendations and the committee's rationale for its recommendations are included in the final report.

As of the date of this CRS report, USDA has not published any rules to amend the WIC food package regulations. As discussed earlier, USDA-FNS regulations based upon scientific recommendations, not the scientific recommendations themselves, govern the program's eligible foods and related issuance policies.

---

[98] Full report, p.29, available at http://nationalacademies.org/hmd/reports/2015/review-wic-food-packages-letterreport.aspx.

[99] http://nationalacademies.org/hmd/reports/2015/review-of-wic-food-packages-interim-report.aspx.

[100] http://nationalacademies.org/hmd/Reports/2017/review-of-wic-food-packages-improving-balance-and-choice.aspx.

APPENDIX C. WIC FARMERS' MARKET NUTRITION PROGRAM (WIC FMNP)

The WIC Farmers' Market Nutrition Program (WIC-FMNP) was first established in 1992.[101] WIC-FMNP provides grants to participating states to offer vouchers/coupons/EBT to WIC participants that may be used in farmers' markets, roadside stands, and other approved venues to purchase fresh produce.[102]

Not all states participate in WIC-FMNP; in FY2015, 38 states, the District of Columbia, 3 U.S. territories, and 6 Indian Tribal Organizations received WIC-FMNP grants.[103] Federal funds primarily cover the program's food costs and 70% of the administrative costs for each participating state. Participating state agencies must provide program income or state, local, or private funds for the program in an amount that is equal to at least 30% of its administrative cost, with some exceptions for tribal agencies.[104]

In FY2015, the program covered an estimated 1.7 million recipients, and about 17,900 farmers, 3,400 farmers' markets, and 2,900 roadside stands. Participants received an average benefit of $23.[105] In FY2015, total WIC-FMNP grant funding was approximately $20 million.[106] FY2016 appropriations (P.L. 114-113) provided $18.5 million for WIC FMNP.

---

[101] WIC-FMNP's authorizing language is at 42 U.S.C. 1786(m). The program was most recently reauthorized by the Healthy, Hunger-Free Kids Act of 2010 (P.L. 111-296).

[102] NOTE: In addition to WIC participants, WIC applicants on a waiting list are also eligible for WIC FMNP. As discussed earlier in this chapter, wait listing has not been necessary in recent years.

[103] USDA-FNS, "WIC FMNP Profiles – Grants and Participation – FY2015," https://www.fns.usda.gov/sites/default/ files/fmnp/FMNP-Profile-Data-FY2015.pdf.

[104] 7 C.F.R. 248.14(a). See also CFDA 10.572.

[105] USDA-FNS, "WIC FMNP Profiles – Grants and Participation – FY2015," https://www.fns.usda.gov/sites/default/ files/fmnp/FMNP-Profile-Data-FY2015.pdf.

[106] See USDA-FNS website for state-specific grant amounts and past years' data, http://www.fns.usda.gov/sites/default/ files/fmnp/WFMNP-Grant-Amounts.pdf.

These are discretionary funds, but while WIC funding is appropriated to the WIC account, WIC-FNMP funds are included in the Commodity Assistance Program account.[107]

---

[107] See generally, President's Budget Justification for USDA-FNS http://www.obpa.usda.gov/32fns2017notes.pdf, pp. 32-74 to 32-90.

In: Child Nutrition Programs
Editor: Daniel D. Coleman
ISBN: 978-1-53615-764-2

Chapter 7

WIC: USDA'S REVIEW OF VEGETABLES AVAILABLE UNDER THE PROGRAM FOLLOWED LEADING RESEARCH PRACTICES*

United States Government Accountability Office

November 30, 2017
Congressional Committees

The Special Supplemental Nutrition Program for Women, Infants, and Children (WIC) provides supplemental foods, nutrition education, including breastfeeding promotion and support, and health and social service program referrals to low-income pregnant, breastfeeding, and postpartum women, infants, and children up to age 5 who are found to be

* This is an edited, reformatted and augmented version of United States Government Accountability Office; Congressional Committees, Publication No. GAO-18-125R, dated November 30, 2017.

at nutritional risk.[1] In fiscal year 2016, WIC provided food and services to about 7.7 million participants, and the federal government spent approximately $6 billion on the program. The U.S. Department of Agriculture's (USDA) Food and Nutrition Service oversees WIC at the federal level and provides grants to state agencies which, in turn, provide food benefits and services to participants through 1,900 local agencies in 10,000 clinic sites.

The federal law authorizing WIC specifies that the supplemental foods provided through the program contain nutrients determined by nutritional research to be lacking in the diets of pregnant, breastfeeding, and postpartum women, infants, and children, and promote the health of the population served by the program. As such, the foods available under WIC are designed to supplement participants' diets with specific nutrients. USDA regulations establish the types and maximum amounts of supplemental food participants may receive. Further, federal law requires USDA to conduct a scientific review of the foods available under WIC at least once every 10 years and amend the foods available, as necessary, to reflect nutrition science, public health concerns, and cultural eating patterns.[2] USDA contracted with the National Academies of Sciences, Engineering, and Medicine (National Academies) for several recent reviews.[3] Among other changes, the 2005 review recommended that fruits and vegetables, with the exception of the white potato, be made available under WIC to better address participants' nutritional needs.[4] The National Academies recommended excluding the white potato based on food intake data for women and young children that showed white potatoes were the

---

[1] WIC is authorized by section 17 of the Child Nutrition Act of 1966, as amended, codified at 42 U.S.C. § 1786. Federal regulations implementing the program may be found at 7 C.F.R. pt. 246.

[2] 42 U.S.C. § 1786(f)(11)(C).

[3] In July 2015, the Institute of Medicine changed its name to the National Academy of Medicine as part of a broad reorganization of the National Academies of Sciences, Engineering, and Medicine (National Academies). The Institute of Medicine is the author of the reports published before that date, and the National Academies is the author of the reports published after that date, although for ease of reference we generally refer only to the National Academies. The mission of the National Academies is to provide independent, objective analysis and advice to inform public policy decisions.

[4] Institute of Medicine, *WIC Food Packages: Time for a Change* (Washington, D.C.: 2005).

most frequently consumed vegetable and average consumption of starchy vegetables met or exceeded recommended amounts.[5] The National Academies' most recent review of WIC foods culminated in three reports, which were issued in 2015 and 2017.[6] The 2015 report that focused on white potatoes recommended that they be available under WIC, in part because nutrients found in white potatoes, such as potassium and fiber, were lacking in WIC participants' diets, and white potatoes can be considered a major source of fiber and other nutrients.[7]

The Consolidated and Further Continuing Appropriations Act of 2015 included a provision for GAO to audit the USDA's most recent review of the supplemental foods available under the program, including the scientific research and data used to conduct USDA's review.[8]

---

[5] Based largely on this recommendation, under an interim rule, USDA allowed fruits and vegetables, except white potatoes, to be purchased with WIC food vouchers in certain WIC food packages, effective October 1, 2009. See Special Supplemental Nutrition Program for Women, Infants and Children (WIC): Revisions in the WIC Food Packages, 72 Fed. Reg. 68,966 (Dec. 6, 2007) and Special Supplemental Nutrition Program for Women, Infants and Children (WIC): Revisions in the WIC Food Packages; Delay of Implementation Date, 73 Fed. Reg. 14,153 (Mar. 17, 2008). The final rule, published in 2014, continued to exclude white potatoes. See Special Supplemental Nutrition Program for Women, Infants and Children (WIC): Revisions in the WIC Food Packages, 79 Fed. Reg. 12,274 (Mar. 4, 2014). The Consolidated and Further Continuing Appropriations Act of 2015 prohibited USDA from using federal funding to exclude or restrict the eligibility of any variety of fresh, whole, or cut vegetables (except for vegetables with added sugars, fats, or oils) from being provided under WIC. The act further directed USDA to commence the next regular review of the supplemental foods available under the program within 90 days of enactment, and provided that the funding restriction would expire if that review concluded that any vegetable shall not be available for purchase under the program, based upon the nutritional content of the vegetable and the nutrition needs of WIC participants. Pub. L. No. 113-235, § 753, 128 Stat. 2130, 2171-72 (2014).

[6] Institute of Medicine, Review of WIC Food Packages: An Evaluation of White Potatoes in the Cash Value Voucher: Letter Report (Washington, D.C.: 2015); National Academies of Sciences, Engineering, and Medicine, Review of WIC Food Packages: Proposed Framework for Revisions: Interim Report (Washington, D.C.: 2015); National Academies of Sciences, Engineering, and Medicine, Review of WIC Food Packages: Improving Balance and Choice: Final Report (Washington, D.C.: 2017). For the purposes of this chapter, we refer to these three reports collectively as "USDA's review."

[7] This chapter also found that because the recommended levels of starchy vegetables had increased, intakes of such vegetables no longer met or exceeded recommended levels; therefore the basis for excluding white potatoes no longer applied.

[8] Pub. L. No. 113-235, § 753(g), 128 Stat. 2130, 2171-72 (2014).

This chapter assesses the extent to which leading research practices were followed in USDA's most recent review of vegetables available under WIC.

To address this objective, we reviewed relevant federal laws, regulations, and guidance, and the three National Academies' reports that comprise USDA's latest review of foods available under WIC. We also reviewed leading research practices identified in our past work, guidance for federal agencies from the Office of Management and Budget (OMB), and reports from other relevant organizations and individuals with expertise in research design (see enclosure I for additional details). For example, the guidance developed by OMB defines professional research principles and practices that should be followed in order to ensure the quality, objectivity, usefulness, and integrity of information disseminated by the federal government. From these sources, we identified eight leading research practices and key components within those practices that are relevant to the three reports that comprise USDA's review of foods available under WIC, and we assessed the extent to which the research conducted for each report followed the identified practices.[9] We also interviewed officials from USDA and the National Academies who were responsible for the recent review of foods available under WIC.

We conducted this performance audit from July 2017 to November 2017 in accordance with generally accepted government auditing standards. Those standards require that we plan and perform the audit to obtain sufficient, appropriate evidence to provide a reasonable basis for our findings and conclusions based on our audit objectives. We believe that the evidence obtained provides a reasonable basis for our findings and conclusions based on our audit objectives.

---

[9] In this chapter, we did not review or assess USDA's contract requirements for the National Academies, USDA's oversight of the contract, or the National Academies' implementation of the contract. Our work focused solely on whether the three resulting reports followed the identified leading research practices.

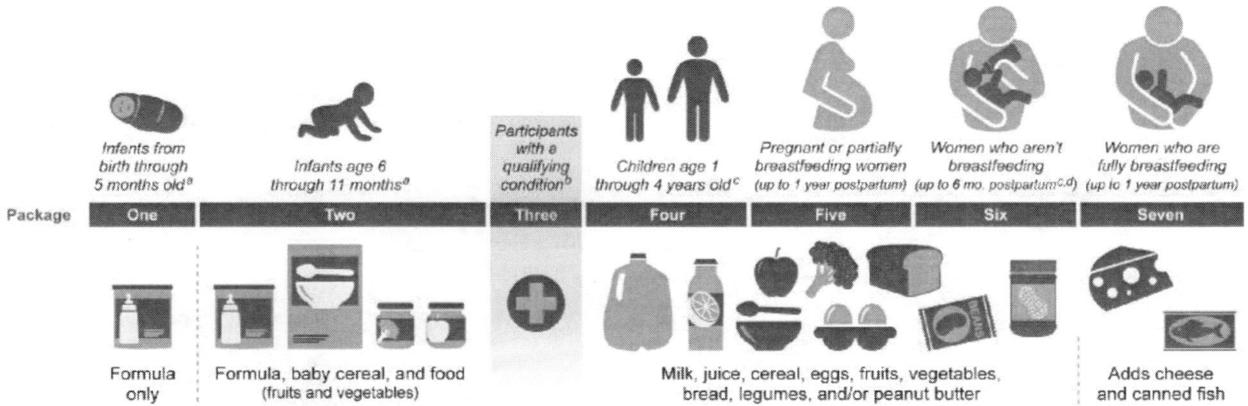

Source: GAO analysis of US Department of Agriculture regulations. GAO-18-125R.

Note: The authorized supplemental foods must be prescribed from food packages according to the category and nutritional needs of the participants. For the complete food package requirements, including which participants are eligible for each package and maximum monthly allowances, see 7 C.F.R. § 246.10(e).

[a]Fully breastfed infants from birth through 5 months do not receive infant formula. Fully breastfed infants age 6 through 11 months may receive meats in addition to baby cereal, fruits, and vegetables; [b]Food Package Three is reserved for participating women, infants, and children with qualifying conditions, such as premature birth, low birth weight, metabolic disorders, gastrointestinal disorders, or immune system disorders. Authorized staff at local agencies determine nutritional risk and prescribe supplemental foods for individuals receiving Food Package Three according to medical documentation provided by health care professionals; [c]Food Packages Four and Six include the option of legumes or peanut butter, but not both. Food Packages Five and Seven include both legumes and peanut butter; [d]Bread is not a category of supplemental food under Food Package Six.

Figure 1. Categories of Foods Available under the Special Supplemental Nutrition Program for Women, Infants and Children (WIC) Food Packages.

BACKGROUND

Established as a national program in the mid-1970s, WIC is intended to improve the health of low-income pregnant and postpartum women, infants, and children by providing supplemental foods, nutrition education, including breastfeeding promotion and support, and referrals to healthcare and social services programs. Pregnant, breastfeeding, and post-partum women, infants, and children under age 5 who are determined to be at nutritional risk and who have incomes below certain thresholds are eligible for WIC. USDA has established seven food packages that are designed for different categories and nutritional needs of WIC participants.[10] Supplemental foods such as vegetables, fruits, cereal, bread, and infant formula may be included in a package (see Figure 1). Families may receive more than one food package if multiple members are eligible to receive WIC benefits. Participants typically receive food benefits in the form of vouchers or checks that they can redeem to obtain approved foods from authorized retailers.[11] The average amount of monthly food benefits provided under WIC was about $43 per participant in fiscal year 2016.

USDA'S REVIEW OF VEGETABLES AVAILABLE UNDER WIC GENERALLY FOLLOWED LEADING RESEARCH PRACTICES FOR DESIGNING STUDIES, IDENTIFYING AND ANALYZING DATA, AND DEVELOPING STATISTICAL ESTIMATES

USDA's review of vegetables available under WIC followed leading research practices for designing studies, according to our analysis of the

[10] 7 C.F.R. § 246.10(e).

[11] In addition, some states issue benefits through a card instead of through paper checks or vouchers in a system called electronic benefit transfer (EBT). State agencies will be required to implement WIC EBT systems by October 1, 2020, unless exempted by USDA. 42 U.S.C. § 1786(h)(12).

three reports that comprise its review (see Figure 2). As we noted in our prior work, evaluations should develop clear and specific research questions and select approaches that enable evaluators to address those questions.[12] In the three reports that comprise USDA's review, which was conducted by the National Academies, the researchers developed clear research questions to examine the food and nutritional needs of the WIC-eligible population. To answer these questions, the researchers used several methodologies and data sources. These included a literature review about diet quality among WIC participants, as well as national survey data on nutrients and types of foods consumed by WIC participants and WIC-eligible nonparticipants, which were compared to levels recommended by the most recent nutritional guidelines.[13] Additionally, the three reports clearly stated limitations in the approaches the researchers used, another research practice we have previously identified as important.[14] For example, the reports noted that the sizes of some subgroups, such as low-income women who were pregnant, were small in the survey data used, and to address this limitation, researchers combined multiple years of data to obtain an adequate number of participants for analysis.

In addition to following leading research practices for designing studies, USDA's review of vegetables available under WIC followed leading practices for identifying and analyzing data, according to our analysis of the three reports that comprise its review (see Figure 3). For example, in the reports, the researchers clearly documented the criteria they used to identify and include studies in the literature review, as well as the databases and search words they used.

---

[12] GAO, *Designing Evaluations: 2012 Revision*, GAO-12-208G (Washington, D.C.: January 2012).

[13] The *Dietary Guidelines for Americans* are nutritional guidelines for the general public. These guidelines are required to be updated by the U.S. Department of Health and Human Services and USDA at least every 5 years based on the preponderance of current scientific and medical knowledge. See 7 U.S.C. § 5341(a). There have been various changes to these guidelines over the years. For example, the most recent guidelines (2015-2020) identified nine nutrients, including potassium, for which many Americans are falling short of recommended amounts.

[14] GAO-12-208G.

Leading Practices	Reports That Comprise USDA's Review of Vegetables Available under WIC Food Packages		
	An Evaluation of White Potatoes[a]	Proposed Framework for Revisions[b]	Improving Balance and Choice[c]
1. Develop useful research questions	●	●	●
a. Are the research questions clear and specific?	☑	☑	☑
b. Do the research questions contain terms that can be readily defined and measured?	☑	☑	☑
c. Are the research questions objective, fair, and neutral?	☑	☑	☑
2. Select methodologies to address the key questions	●	●	●
a. Does the study methodology address all key questions?	☑	☑	☑
b. Does the study methodology provide the precision, completeness, and conclusiveness of the information needed to answer the questions?	☑	☑	☑
3. Select data sources to address key questions	●	●	●
a. Is the data free of bias or other significant errors that could lead to inaccurate conclusions?	☑	☑	☑
b. Is the data sufficient to persuade a knowledgeable person that the findings are reasonable?	☑	☑	☑
c. Is the data relevant, valid, and reliable?	☑	☑	☑
4. Document methodologies and limitations	●	●	●
a. Does the study describe the data sources used?	☑	☑	☑
b. Does the study document assumptions and procedures?	☑	☑	☑
c. Are limitations clearly stated about what the study can and cannot address?	☑	☑	☑
d. Are the strengths and weaknesses that are embedded in the methodology clearly stated?	☑	☑	☑

● = Followed ☑ = Yes

Note: The leading research practices identified in this figure are based on guidance for federal agencies from the Office of Management and Budget and reports from other relevant organizations and individuals with expertise in research design.

[a]Institute of Medicine, Review of WIC Food Packages: An Evaluation of White Potatoes in the Cash Value Voucher: Letter Report (Washington, D.C.: 2015).

[b]National Academies of Sciences, Engineering, and Medicine, Review of WIC Food Packages: Proposed Framework for Revisions: Interim Report (Washington, D.C.: 2015).

[c]National Academies of Sciences, Engineering, and Medicine, Review of WIC Food Packages: Improving Balance and Choice: Final Report (Washington, D.C.: 2017).

Figure 2. GAO Analysis of the Extent to Which USDA's Review of Vegetables Available under the Special Supplemental Nutrition Program for Women, Infants, and Children (WIC) Followed Leading Practices for Designing Studies.

Leading Practices	Reports That Comprise USDA's Review of Vegetables Available under WIC Food Packages: An Evaluation of White Potatoes[a]	Proposed Framework for Revisions[b]	Improving Balance and Choice[c]
1. Developing literature reviews	Followed	Followed	Followed
a. Does the literature review clearly state its criteria?	Yes	Yes	Yes
b. Were the studies in the literature review assessed for their strengths and weaknesses?	Yes	Yes	Yes
2. Developing statistical estimates	Partially followed	Followed	Followed
a. Are sufficient steps taken to make estimates to a larger population (i.e., the overall population of individuals to which the conclusions are to be applied)?	Yes	Yes	Yes
b. Are estimates based on generally accepted methods (e.g., sampling errors that are associated with the estimates due to sampling some but not all of the individuals)?	No	Yes	Yes
3. Making comparisons	Did not follow	Followed	Followed
a. Does study test and report only the differences that are statistically significant (i.e., differences that are not a result of chance alone)?	No	Yes	Yes
4. Developing economic analysis	Followed	Followed	Followed
a. Does economic analysis include a statement of what action is being examined and the timeframe of the analysis?	Yes	Yes	Yes
b. Does economic analysis identify alternatives (e.g., analysis of change compared to no change)?	Yes	Yes	Yes
c. Does analysis include economic effects?	Yes	Yes	Yes
d. Does economic analysis include a sensitivity analysis (i.e., how possible changes impact the outcome)?	Yes	Yes	Yes
e. Does the economic analysis include adequate documentation and transparency (e.g. cites data sources, discloses limitations and contributors, etc.)?	Yes	Yes	Yes

● = Followed ◐ = Partially followed ○ = Did not follow ☑ = Yes ☐ = No

Source: GAO analysis of studies conducted by National Academies of Sciences, Engineering, and Medicine for the U.S. Department of Agriculture. GAO-18-125R.

Note: The leading research practices identified in this figure are based on guidance for federal agencies from the Office of Management and Budget and reports from other relevant organizations and individuals with expertise in research design.

[a]Institute of Medicine, Review of WIC Food Packages: An Evaluation of White Potatoes in the Cash Value Voucher: Letter Report (Washington, D.C.: 2015).

[b]National Academies of Sciences, Engineering, and Medicine, Review of WIC Food Packages: Proposed Framework for Revisions: Interim Report (Washington, D.C.: 2015).

[c]National Academies of Sciences, Engineering, and Medicine, Review of WIC Food Packages: Improving Balance and Choice: Final Report (Washington, D.C.: 2017).

Figure 3. GAO Analysis of the Extent to Which USDA's Review of Vegetables Available under the Special Supplemental Nutrition Program for Women, Infants, and Children (WIC) Followed Leading Practices for Identifying and Analyzing Data.

Further, OMB guidance notes that agencies should take sufficient steps to develop statistical estimates that apply to a larger population, not just the subset of individuals for which they have information.[15] Such steps may include adjusting an agency's analysis to more accurately reflect the general population. In the three reports that comprise USDA's review, researchers followed this leading practice. For example, in their analysis of the National Health and Nutrition Examination Survey (NHANES), they developed statistical estimates that applied to WIC participants generally, not just those who were part of the survey.[16] We also found that all three reports followed leading research practices for developing economic analyses. For example, the researchers analyzed the costs of the current foods available under WIC and compared those to various alternatives.

USDA's review of vegetables available under WIC also generally followed leading practices for developing statistical estimates and making comparisons between subgroups. OMB guidance recommends that agencies should provide additional information about the range of possible estimates that may also be valid due to selecting some but not all individuals in a population. As previously noted, for the reports that comprise USDA's review, the researchers used food consumption data obtained from NHANES, which gathered information from a subset of individuals. From these data, statistical estimates were made that were relevant to a larger population. However, NHANES gathered information from one of multiple possible subsets of relevant individuals, and each of these subsets could have produced different estimates. Leading research practices indicate that this variation in possible estimates should be noted, such as by indicating upper and lower bounds on each estimate.[17] Such

---

[15] Office of Management and Budget, *Standards and Guidelines for Statistical Surveys* (Washington, D.C.: September 2006).

[16] NHANES is a survey conducted by the Centers for Disease Control and Prevention that consists of questionnaires as well as a standardized health examination. It provides information on the health and nutritional status of adults and children in the United States.

[17] Additional information on the variation in possible estimates may be presented as upper and lower bounds, standard errors, or margin of errors. For example, an estimate for one sample may be 56 percent while estimates for different samples from the same population might be 50 percent, 55 percent, 60 percent or 62 percent. For the 56 percent estimate, a leading research practice is to note that it has a margin of error of plus or minus 6 percent with a lower bound of 50 percent and an upper bound of 62 percent.

information is included in two of the three reports that comprise USDA's recent review of foods available under WIC, but it is not included in the 2015 report on the white potato. An official from the National Academies told us that this information was not included because it was not requested in USDA's technical proposal for that study. Similarly, the 2015 report on the white potato did not include sufficient information for making comparisons between relevant subgroups. OMB guidance notes that agencies should provide information on the significance of differences between subgroups.[18] As previously noted, all three reports provided estimates on nutritional intake for WIC participants and eligible non-participants. However, the 2015 report on the white potato did not include the additional information necessary to determine if differences in the estimates for the subgroups were significant.[19] The report notes that, for some of the subgroups, the sample sizes were too small to make statistical comparisons.

Agency Comments

We provided a draft of this chapter to USDA for review and comment. USDA provided technical comments, which we incorporated as appropriate.

We are sending copies of this chapter to the appropriate congressional committees and the Secretary of the U.S. Department of Agriculture.

Kathryn Larin
Director, Education, Workforce, and Income Security

---

[18] Specifically, this guidance states that agencies should report only the differences that are large enough to be substantively meaningful, even if other differences are also statistically significant.

[19] Although this information would have been useful in determining the extent diets differ between WIC participants and WIC-eligible nonparticipants, the evaluation found that both of these groups have inadequate levels of certain nutrients, such as potassium and fiber, and that some of these nutrients are provided by the white potato.

Nancy Kingsbury
Managing Director, Applied Research and Methods

List of Committees

The Honorable Pat Roberts
Chairman

The Honorable Debbie Stabenow
Ranking Member
Committee on Agriculture, Nutrition, and Forestry
United States Senate

The Honorable John Hoeven
Chairman

The Honorable Jeff Merkley
Ranking Member
Subcommittee on Agriculture, Rural Development,
Food and Drug Administration, and Related Agencies
Committee on Appropriations
United States Senate

The Honorable Virginia Foxx
Chair

The Honorable Robert C. "Bobby" Scott
Ranking Member
Committee on Education and the Workforce
House of Representatives

The Honorable Robert Aderholt
Chairman

The Honorable Sanford Bishop
Ranking Member
Subcommittee on Agriculture, Rural Development,
Food and Drug Administration, and Related Agencies
Committee on Appropriations
House of Representatives

In: Child Nutrition Programs
Editor: Daniel D. Coleman
ISBN: 978-1-53615-764-2

Chapter 8

SUPPLEMENTAL NUTRITION ASSISTANCE PROGRAM: OBSERVATIONS ON EMPLOYMENT AND TRAINING PROGRAMS AND EFFORTS TO ADDRESS PROGRAM INTEGRITY ISSUES*

Kathryn Larin

WHY GAO DID THIS STUDY

SNAP is the largest federally funded nutrition assistance program. In fiscal year 2017, it provided about $63 billion in benefits. USDA and the states jointly administer SNAP and partner to address issues that affect program integrity, including improper payments and fraud. GAO has

* This is an edited, reformatted and augmented version of United States Government Accountability Office, Testimony Before the Subcommittees on, Healthcare, Benefits and Administrative, Rules and Intergovernmental Affairs, Committee on Oversight and Government Reform, House of Representatives, Publication No. GAO-18-504T, dated May 9, 2018.

previously reported on various aspects of SNAP, including state SNAP E&T programs, improper payment rates, recipient fraud, and retailer trafficking.

This testimony discusses GAO's prior and ongoing work on (1) SNAP E&T programs, including program participants, design, and USDA oversight, and (2) USDA's efforts to address SNAP program integrity, including improper payments, as well as recipient and retailer fraud. As part of its ongoing work on SNAP E&T programs, GAO analyzed E&T expenditures and participation data from fiscal years 2007 through 2016, the most recent data available; reviewed relevant research from USDA; and interviewed USDA and selected state and local officials. The prior work discussed in this testimony is based on four GAO products on E&T programs (GAO-03-388), improper payments (GAO-16-708T), recipient fraud (GAO-14-641), and retailer trafficking (GAO-07-53). Information on the scope and methodology of our prior work is available in each product.

What GAO Recommends

GAO is not making new recommendations. USDA generally concurred with GAO's prior recommendations.

What GAO Found

Overseen by the U.S. Department of Agriculture (USDA) and administered by states, Supplemental Nutrition Assistance Program (SNAP) Employment and Training (E&T) programs served about 0.5 percent of the approximately 43.5 million SNAP recipients in an average month of fiscal year 2016, according to the most recent USDA data available. These programs are generally designed to help SNAP recipients increase their ability to obtain regular employment through services such as job search and training. Some recipients may be required to participate.

According to USDA, about 14 percent of SNAP recipients were subject to work requirements in an average month of fiscal year 2016, while others, such as children and the elderly, were generally exempt from these requirements. States have flexibility in how they design their E&T programs. Over the last several years, states have 1) increasingly moved away from programs that mandate participation, 2) focused on serving able-bodied adults without dependents whose benefits are generally time-limited unless they comply with work requirements, and 3) partnered with state and local organizations to deliver services. USDA has taken steps to increase support and oversight of SNAP E&T since 2014, including collecting new data on participant outcomes from states. GAO has ongoing work reviewing SNAP E&T programs, including USDA oversight.

USDA and the states partner to address issues that affect program integrity, including improper payments and fraud, and USDA has taken some steps to address challenges in these areas, but issues remain.

- Improper Payments. In 2016, GAO reviewed SNAP improper payment rates and found that states' adoption of program flexibilities and changes in federal SNAP policy in the previous decade, as well as improper payment rate calculation methods, likely affected these rates. Although USDA reported improper payment estimates for SNAP in previous years, USDA did not report an estimate for benefits paid in fiscal years 2015 or 2016 due to data quality issues in some states. USDA has since been working with the states to improve improper payment estimates for the fiscal year 2017 review.
- Recipient Fraud. In 2014, GAO made recommendations to USDA to address challenges states faced in combatting recipient fraud. For example, GAO found that USDA's guidance on the use of transaction data to uncover potential trafficking lacked specificity and recommended USDA develop additional guidance. Since then, USDA has provided technical assistance to some states, including on the use of data analytics. GAO has ongoing work reviewing states' use of data analytics to identify SNAP recipient fraud.

- Retailer Trafficking. In 2006, GAO identified several ways in which SNAP was vulnerable to retailer trafficking—a practice involving the exchange of benefits for cash or non-food items. For example, USDA had not conducted analyses to identify high-risk retailers and target its resources. Since then, USDA has established risk levels for retailers based on various factors. GAO has ongoing work assessing how USDA prevents, detects, and responds to retailer trafficking and reviewing the usefulness of USDA's estimates of the extent of SNAP retailer trafficking.

Chairman Jordan, Chairman Palmer, Ranking Member Krishnamoorthi, Ranking Member Raskin, and Members of the Subcommittees:

Thank you for inviting me here today to discuss our work on the U.S. Department of Agriculture's (USDA) Supplemental Nutrition Assistance Program (SNAP)—the largest federally-funded nutrition assistance program. Jointly administered by USDA's Food and Nutrition Service (FNS) and the states, SNAP helps low-income households obtain a better diet by providing them with benefits to purchase food from authorized retailers. In fiscal year 2017, SNAP provided approximately $63 billion in benefits to about 42 million individuals in over 20 million households.

To receive SNAP benefits, individuals must apply in their state of residence and meet the program's eligibility requirements, such as income limits. To be eligible for benefits, SNAP recipients must also generally comply with the program's work requirements, such as registering for work and participating in certain work programs if required by the state agency.[1] For example, SNAP recipients may be required by the state to participate in state-operated SNAP Employment and Training (E&T) programs. First federally required in the 1980s, SNAP E&T programs are

[1] The general SNAP work requirements apply to people ages 16 through 59, except for those who are physically or mentally unfit, have responsibility for the care of a dependent child under age 6 or an incapacitated person, are already employed 30 hours or more per week or receive weekly earnings which equal the minimum hourly rate set under federal law multiplied by 30, or are a bona fide student enrolled half-time or more in any recognized school training program, or institution of higher education, amongst other exceptions.

intended to help individuals in SNAP households acquire skills, training, employment, or experience that will increase their ability to obtain regular employment.

The federal government pays the full cost of SNAP benefits and shares the costs and responsibility of administering the program and ensuring program integrity with the states. Most SNAP benefits are used for the intended purpose, according to FNS. However, improper payments—payments to individuals that were made in an incorrect amount of should not have been made at all—may result from unintentional errors by SNAP recipients or staff administering the program or may result from intentional errors or misuse of benefits, practices which are considered fraud. For example, individuals may misrepresent their household's circumstances to state agencies in order to obtain benefits. Further, some recipients sell their benefits for cash, often at a loss, to a retailer—a practice known as trafficking. FNS is responsible for authorizing and monitoring retailers from which recipients may purchase food, and states are responsible for determining applicant eligibility and investigating possible program violations by recipients. As we have reported in our prior work, both FNS and states face challenges in addressing recipient and retailer fraud.

In response to requests from the Chairman and other members of this Committee, we currently have work underway on SNAP E&T programs, as well as on SNAP recipient and retailer fraud. Today I will provide information from our ongoing and prior work, focusing on (1) SNAP E&T programs, including program participants, design, and FNS oversight, and (2) FNS's efforts to address program integrity, including improper payments and SNAP recipient and retailer fraud.

To address the areas discussed in this testimony statement, we drew on our ongoing work on SNAP E&T programs, recipient fraud, retailer trafficking, as well as our prior work on improper payments. Specifically, for our discussion of SNAP E&T programs, we analyzed data on SNAP E&T expenditures and participation collected by FNS from the states for fiscal year 2007 through fiscal year 2016, the most recent data available. In addition, we analyzed published FNS Quality Control data on SNAP recipients and work registrants for fiscal year 2008 through fiscal year

2016. To assess the reliability of the data included in this statement, we interviewed FNS and state officials knowledgeable about the data, and determined the data are sufficiently reliable for the purposes of this statement. We also reviewed relevant federal laws and regulations; reviewed guidance and research from FNS; interviewed FNS officials, as well as select state and local SNAP E&T staff from five states; and reviewed our prior work on SNAP E&T programs.[2] For our discussion of FNS's efforts to address improper payments and SNAP recipient and retailer fraud, we drew on our 2016 review of SNAP improper payment rates and reviewed relevant USDA reports.[3] We also drew on our 2014 analysis of SNAP replacement card and transaction data, in which we conducted tests of FNS-recommended automated tools and interviewed program stakeholders, including federal and select state officials.[4] We also obtained relevant documentation from FNS in April 2018 on steps the agency has taken to address our 2014 recommendations. We also drew on our 2006 work on retailer trafficking, in which we reviewed FNS reports on trafficking estimates; visited FNS field offices; analyzed FNS retailer data; and interviewed federal officials, among others.[5] We also assessed FNS reports on trafficking estimates covering calendar years 2006 through 2014 (the most recent data available), reviewed FNS policies and reports, and interviewed FNS officials.[6] More complete information on the scope and methodology of our prior work is available in each published report.

---

[2] In our ongoing work, we selected states based on several criteria, including varied SNAP E&T service delivery approaches and other program characteristics, as well as geographic dispersion. Our prior work on SNAP E&T is included in our 2003 report: GAO, *Food Stamp Employment and Training Program: Better Data Needed to Understand Who Is Served and What the Program Achieves*. GAO-03-388. (Washington, D.C.: March 12, 2003).

[3] GAO, *Supplemental Nutrition Assistance Program: Policy Changes and Calculation Methods Likely Affect Improper Payment Rates, and USDA Is Taking Steps to Help Address Recipient Fraud*, GAO-16-708T (Washington, D.C.: July 6, 2016).

[4] GAO, *Supplemental Nutrition Assistance Program: Enhanced Detection Tools and Reporting Could Improve Efforts to Combat Recipient Fraud*, GAO-14-641. (Washington, D.C.: August 21, 2014).

[5] GAO, *Food Stamp Trafficking: FNS Could Enhance Program Integrity by Better Targeting Stores Likely to Traffic and Increasing Penalties*. GAO-07-53. (Washington, D.C.: Oct. 13, 2006).

[6] FNS's *The Extent of Trafficking in the Supplemental Nutrition Assistance Program* reports are published approximately two to three years after the time period covered in the report. For example, the most recent report—published in 2017—analyzes data from 2012 to 2014.

Our current work on SNAP E&T programs, recipient fraud, and retailer trafficking is still ongoing.

The work upon which this statement is based was conducted in accordance with generally accepted government auditing standards. Those standards require that we plan and perform the audit to obtain sufficient, appropriate evidence to provide a reasonable basis for our findings and conclusions based on our audit objectives. We believe that the evidence obtained provides a reasonable basis for our findings and conclusions based on our audit objectives.

BACKGROUND

USDA's Food and Nutrition Service (FNS) is responsible for promulgating SNAP program regulations, ensuring that state officials administer the program in compliance with program rules, and authorizing and monitoring retailers from which recipients may purchase food. States are responsible for determining applicant eligibility, calculating the amount of their benefits, issuing benefits on Electronic Benefit Transfer (EBT) cards—which can be used like debit cards to purchase food from authorized retailers—and investigating possible program violations by recipients.

SNAP Work Requirements

SNAP recipients are subject to various work requirements. Generally, all SNAP recipients ages 16 through 59, unless exempted by law or regulation, must comply with work requirements, including registering for work, reporting to an employer if referred by a state agency, accepting a bona fide offer of a suitable job, not voluntarily quitting a job or reducing work hours below 30 hours a week, and participating in a SNAP E&T program or a workfare program—in which recipients perform work on behalf of the state—if assigned by the state agency.[7] SNAP recipients are generally exempt from complying with these work requirements if they are physically or mentally unfit, responsible for caring for a dependent child under age 6 or an incapacitated person, employed for 30 or more hours per week or receive weekly earnings which equal the minimum hourly rate set under federal law multiplied by 30, or are a bona fide student enrolled half-time or more in any recognized school training program, or institution of higher education, amongst other exemptions. SNAP recipients subject to the work requirements—known as work registrants— may lose their eligibility for benefits if they fail to comply with these requirements without good cause.[8]

One segment of the work registrant population, SNAP recipients ages 18 through 49 who are "able-bodied," not responsible for a dependent child, and do not meet other exemptions—able-bodied adults without dependents (ABAWDs)—are generally subject to additional work requirements. In addition to meeting the general work requirements, ABAWDs must work or participate in a work program 20 hours or more per week, or participate in workfare, in which ABAWDs perform work to earn the value of their SNAP benefits. Participation in SNAP E&T, which is a type of work program, is one way for ABAWDs to meet the 20 hour per week ABAWD work requirement, but other work programs are acceptable as well. Unless ABAWDs meet these work requirements or are determined to be exempt, they are limited to 3 months of SNAP benefits in a 36-month period.[9]

At the request of states, FNS may waive the ABAWD time limit for ABAWDs located in certain areas of a state or an entire state under certain

---

[7] Regarding work registration, SNAP recipients subject to work requirements are required to register for work or be registered by the state agency at the time of application and every 12 months after initial registration.

[8] Examples of good cause can include illness, household emergency, lack of transportation, and other circumstances. States must determine if a recipient has good cause for not complying with work requirements before disqualifying the recipient from benefits.

[9] According to FNS, reasons for ABAWD exemptions may include medically certified as physically or mentally unfit for employment, responsible for a child under 18, employed for 30 or more hours per week, or pregnant. Further, state agencies have discretion to exempt, on a month-to-month basis, 15 percent of the ABAWDs who would otherwise be subject to the time limit.

circumstances. A waiver may be granted if the area has an unemployment rate of over 10 percent or there are an insufficient number of jobs to provide employment for these individuals. If the time limit is waived, ABAWDs are not required to meet the ABAWD work requirement in order to receive SNAP for more than 3 months in a 36-month period yet they must still comply with the general work requirements.

SNAP Employment and Training Programs

Federal requirements for state SNAP E&T programs were first enacted in 1985 and provide state SNAP agencies with flexibility in how they design their SNAP E&T programs, including who to serve and what services to offer. The state has the option to offer SNAP E&T services on a voluntary basis to some or all SNAP recipients, an approach commonly referred to as a voluntary program. Alternatively, the state can require some or all SNAP work registrants to participate in the SNAP E&T program as a condition of eligibility, an approach commonly referred to as a mandatory program. Further, states determine which service components to provide participants through their SNAP E&T programs, although they must provide at least one from a federally determined list. This list includes job search programs, job search training programs, workfare, programs designed to improve employability through work experience or training, education programs to improve basic skills and employability, job retention services, and programs to improve self-sufficiency through self-employment. Total federal expenditures on SNAP E&T programs were more than $337 million in fiscal year 2016. States are eligible to receive three types of federal funding available for state SNAP E&T programs: 100 percent funds—formula grants for program administration,[10] 50

[10] Federal 100 percent funds are set at $90 million by statute. Federal 100 percent funds are allocated to states based on a formula, in which 90 percent of the state's allocation is based on the number of work registrants in a state and 10 percent of the allocation is based on the number of ABAWDs in a state.

percent federal reimbursement funds, and ABAWD pledge funds—grants to states that pledge to serve all of their at-risk ABAWDs.[11]

SNAP Program Integrity

The Office of Management and Budget has designated SNAP as a high-priority program due to the estimated dollar amount in improper payments—any payments that should not have been made or were made in an incorrect amount (including overpayments and underpayments) under statutory, contractual, administrative, or other legally applicable requirements. According to USDA's fiscal year 2015 agency financial report, $2.6 billion, or 3.66 percent, of all SNAP benefits paid in fiscal year 2014 were improper, the most recent year for which data are available. SNAP improper payments are caused by variances in any of the key factors involved in determining SNAP eligibility and benefit amounts, and, according to USDA, household income was the most common primary cause of dollar errors.[12] States review the accuracy of SNAP payments to recipients on an ongoing basis, and FNS assesses the accuracy of state reviews and determines a national improper payment rate annually.

FNS and states share responsibility for addressing SNAP fraud, which can occur through the eligibility process and when benefits are being used.

---

[11] ABAWD pledge funds are set at not more than $20 million by statute. States receiving ABAWD pledge funds from the federal government must make and comply with a commitment, or pledge, to use these funds to offer at-risk ABAWDs a position in an education, training or workforce component that fulfills the ABAWD work requirement. At-risk ABAWDs are those in the last month of the three month time limit of SNAP eligibility and who meet other criteria. The ABAWD grants are allocated based on the number of ABAWDs in the states participating in the pledge. States may also use the other SNAP E&T funding streams to serve ABAWDs.

[12] FNS developed its quality control process for SNAP in 1977 to track and measure errors in both eligibility and benefit determinations for the program. According to FNS officials, each month, a state's SNAP quality control staff selects for review a representative sample of households that received SNAP benefits. The statewide sample is designed to produce a valid statewide improper payment rate, which is the sum of the overpayments and underpayments divided by the value of all payments. A variance occurs when a quality control reviewer finds the incorrect application of policy, the basis of issuance is incorrect, or there is a difference between the information that was used and the information that should have been used to determine a household's monthly SNAP benefit amount.

Specifically, recipients may commit eligibility fraud when they misrepresent their household size, income, or expenses in order to fraudulently obtain SNAP benefits. Another type of fraud—trafficking—occurs when recipients exchange benefits with authorized retailers or other individuals for cash or non-food items (e.g., rent or transportation). In a typical retailer trafficking situation, for example, a retailer may charge $100 to a recipient's EBT card and give the recipient $50 in cash instead of $100 in food. The federal government reimburses the retailer $100, which results in a fraudulent $50 profit to the retailer.

State agencies are directly responsible for preventing, detecting, investigating, and prosecuting recipient fraud, including eligibility fraud and trafficking by SNAP recipients, under the oversight and guidance of FNS. States play a key role in preventing fraud when determining eligibility for SNAP. State agencies collect applicant information, such as household income and employment, and verify it through data matches with other information sources. After benefits are issued, the agencies may monitor EBT transaction data to identify spending patterns that may indicate trafficking. If an individual or household intentionally violates SNAP rules, such as by trafficking or making false or misleading statements in order to obtain benefits, states conduct administrative disqualification hearings or, in some cases, refer the case for criminal prosecution.

FNS is responsible for authorizing and overseeing retailers who participate in the program—totaling more than 263,000 in fiscal year 2017—including investigating potential retailer trafficking. In order to participate in SNAP, a retailer applies to FNS and demonstrates that they meet program requirements, such as those on the amount and types of food that authorized stores must carry. FNS verifies a retailer's compliance with these requirements and generally authorizes retailers for 5 years. FNS then monitors retailers' continued compliance with program requirements and administratively disqualifies, or assesses money penalties on, those who are found to have trafficked benefits. To this end, FNS officials collect and monitor EBT transaction data to detect irregular patterns of transactions that may indicate trafficking and also conduct undercover investigations. If found to be trafficking, retailers are generally permanently disqualified from SNAP or incur a monetary penalty in lieu of permanent disqualification.[13]

A Small Percentage of SNAP Recipients Participate in SNAP E&T Programs, Which Have Experienced Changes in Characteristics and FNS Oversight

A Small Percentage of SNAP Recipients Participate in SNAP E&T

According to FNS data, about 14 percent of SNAP recipients, or about 6.1 million, were work registrants who were subject to work requirements,[14] and about 0.5 percent of SNAP recipients, or about 200,000, participated in state SNAP E&T programs, in an average month of fiscal year 2016.[15] (See Figure 1.) According to FNS, most SNAP recipients are exempt from work requirements. For example, according to FNS, almost two-thirds of SNAP recipients were children, elderly, or adults with a disability in an average month of fiscal year 2016—groups that are generally exempt. Further, adults who are already working at least

---

[13] The retailer may appeal FNS's decision, first within FNS and later to the appropriate federal district court. The USDA Office of Inspector General, U.S. Secret Service, and the Federal Bureau of Investigation also conduct investigations of SNAP retailers, which may lead to criminal prosecutions.

[14] Estimates for SNAP recipients overall and work registrants are FNS estimates derived from a monthly sample of SNAP households. We have not yet assessed the statistical precision of these estimates or whether changes over time and among subgroups of recipients are statistically significant. We plan to further assess these estimates as part of our ongoing work.

[15] The average monthly SNAP recipients and work registrants in the fiscal year 2016 SNAP Quality Control data are derived from an independent monthly sample of participating SNAP households selected from October 2015 through September 2016. To calculate the average monthly number of SNAP recipients participating in SNAP E&T programs, we calculated the total number of recipients participating in SNAP E&T components across all months in fiscal year 2016 and divided by 12.

30 hours a week are also exempt from SNAP work requirements, and according to FNS data, more than 31 percent of non-elderly adult SNAP recipients were employed in an average month of fiscal year 2016.[16] SNAP work registrants who are not participating in SNAP E&T programs may be participating in other activities to meet work requirements or eligible for other exemptions.[17] FNS officials told us that the state data reported to FNS on SNAP E&T participants are the best and most recent data available on this group, yet they also have limitations, which we will continue to explore in our ongoing work.[18]

In recent years, the number and percentage of SNAP recipients and work registrants participating in SNAP E&T programs appears to have decreased, according to FNS data. From fiscal year 2008 through fiscal year 2016, the average monthly number of SNAP E&T participants decreased from about 256,000 to about 207,000, or by 19 percent, according to state data on SNAP E&T participants reported to FNS. (See Figure 2.) However, over the same time period, the average monthly number of SNAP recipients appears to have increased from about 27.8 million to about 43.5 million, and work registrants appears to have increased from about 3 million to about 6.1 million, according to FNS data. As a result, the percentage of total SNAP recipients participating in SNAP E&T programs decreased from about 0.9 to about 0.5 percent, and the percentage of SNAP work registrants participating in these programs decreased from approximately 8.1 percent to 3.4 percent, from fiscal year 2008 through fiscal year 2016.[19]

---

[16] This includes employed adults with a disability.

[17] There are other federal exemptions from SNAP work requirements, such as having responsibility for caring for a dependent child under six or an incapacitated person, or complying with work requirements for certain other programs, such as Temporary Assistance for Needy Families.

[18] According to FNS, state data on SNAP E&T participants have various limitations, in part because the data are state-reported and not subject to multiple verification processes. FNS officials noted that some of the common reporting errors made by states result in inconsistencies between quarterly and annual reports, incorrect reporting of ABAWDs, duplicate counts of SNAP E&T participants, and undercounts or duplicate counts of work registrants, among others. We are continuing to examine these data limitations as part of our ongoing work.

[19] According to FNS officials, some SNAP recipients who are exempt from work registration requirements may participate in SNAP E&T programs, yet there are no data available which

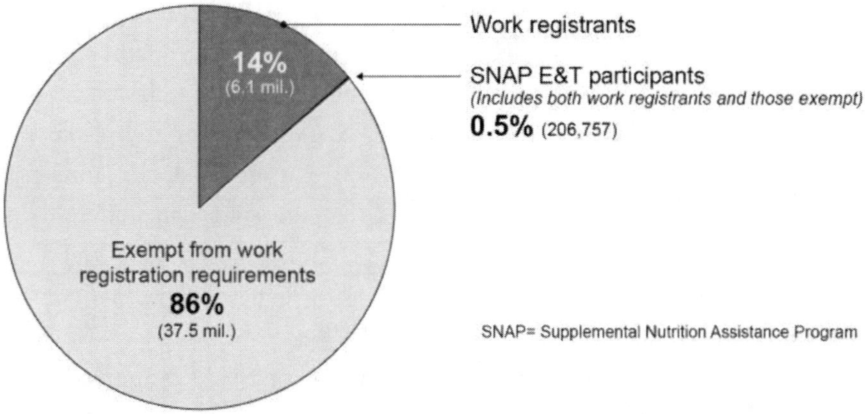

Source: GAO analysis of Food and Nutrition Service SNAP Quality Control and from 583 data. | GAO-18-504T.

Note: Data include the 50 states, District of Columbia, Guam, and the Virgin Islands. According to FNS officials, available data on SNAP E&T participants have certain limitations, given that the data are state-reported and not subject to multiple verification processes. According to FNS officials, some SNAP recipients who are exempt from work registration requirements may participate in SNAP E&T programs, yet there are no data available which would allow us to calculate how many such recipients do so. Estimates for SNAP recipients overall and work registrants are FNS estimates derived from a monthly sample of SNAP households. We have not yet assessed the statistical precision of these estimates or whether changes over time and among subgroups of recipients are statistically significant. We plan to further assess these estimates as part of our ongoing work.

Figure 1. Average Monthly State SNAP Employment and Training (E&T) Program Participants as a Percentage of Average Monthly SNAP Recipients, Fiscal Year 2016.

Available information suggests the characteristics of SNAP E&T participants are generally similar to those of SNAP work registrants who do not participate in these programs.

---

would allow us to calculate how many such recipients do so. As a result, these percentages may overstate the percentage of work registrants participating in SNAP E&T programs.

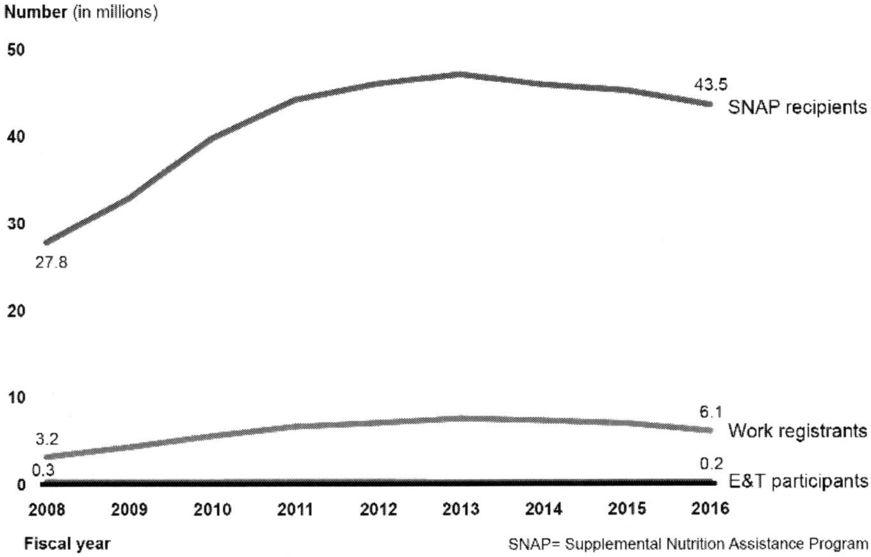

Source: GAO analysis of Food and Nutrition Service SNAP Quality Control and from 583 data. | GAO-18-504T.

Note: Data include the 50 states, District of Columbia, Guam, and the Virgin Islands. According to FNS officials, available data on SNAP E&T participants have certain limitations, given that the data are state-reported and not subject to multiple verification processes. According to FNS officials, some SNAP recipients who are exempt from work registration requirements may participate in SNAP E&T programs, yet there are no data available which would allow us to calculate how many such recipients do so. As a result, these percentages may overstate the percentage of work registrants participating in SNAP E&T programs. Estimates for SNAP recipients overall and work registrants are FNS estimates derived from a monthly sample of SNAP households. We have not yet assessed the statistical precision of these estimates or whether changes over time and among subgroups of recipients are statistically significant. We plan to further assess these estimates as part of our ongoing work.

Figure 2. Average Monthly Federal SNAP Employment and Training (E&T) Participants Compared with Average Monthly Work Registrants and SNAP Recipients, Fiscal Years 2008 to 2016.

A recent FNS study, which surveyed SNAP E&T participants and SNAP work registrants who had not participated in SNAP E&T, found that members of the two groups had similar demographic characteristics, including age and gender, and received similar monthly SNAP benefit amounts.[20] Further, at the time they were surveyed, about one third of each group were employed, and their average wage rates were similar, at about $10 per hour.[21]

State SNAP E&T Programs Have Changed in Several Ways

State SNAP agencies have broad flexibility in how they design their SNAP E&T programs, and the characteristics of these programs have changed in several ways over the last decade. For example, states have increasingly moved from mandatory to voluntary programs, focused on serving ABAWDs, and partnered with state and local organizations to deliver services.

States Have Increasingly Moved from Mandatory to Voluntary Programs

According to FNS data, states have increasingly moved from mandatory to voluntary SNAP E&T programs in recent years.[22] In fiscal year 2010, 17 states operated voluntary programs; however, by fiscal year 2017, 35 states operated voluntary programs, according to FNS data (See Figure 3). FNS officials told us that they have been actively encouraging states to provide more robust employment and training services, such as vocational training or work experience, through voluntary programs. They said that they believe these types of robust services are more effective in

---

[20] Rowe, Gretchen, Elizabeth Brown, and Brian Estes. *SNAP Employment and Training (E&T) Characteristics Study: Final Report.* Prepared by Mathematica Policy Research for the U.S. Department of Agriculture, Food and Nutrition Service, Oct. 2017.

[21] The survey was conducted several months after respondents were identified as work registrants or SNAP E&T participants. Their circumstances could have changed during this period, including completing an SNAP E&T program and finding full-time employment. Although working more than 30 hours a week is an exemption from SNAP work requirements, study authors state that a number of the respondents might have been designated as work registrants many months prior to the survey. In addition, SNAP E&T participants included those who had participated in the program within the previous 24 months and might have become employed after completion of the SNAP E&T program.

[22] FNS categorizes state SNAP E&T programs as either mandatory or voluntary. Some states operate mandatory SNAP E&T programs in certain localities rather than statewide. These states are denoted as having mandatory programs.

moving participants toward self-sufficiency, but that funding may not be sufficient to provide these to the large numbers of participants served in mandatory programs. In addition, FNS officials told us that voluntary programs are less administratively burdensome than mandatory programs, as they allow states to focus on serving motivated participants rather than sanctioning non-compliant individuals.

According to FNS officials, when states move to a voluntary program, they generally experience a decline in SNAP E&T participation—a trend consistent with our analysis of FNS data—which may have contributed to the decline in overall SNAP E&T participation. Of the 22 states or territories that changed from a mandatory to a voluntary program from fiscal year 2010 through fiscal year 2016, according to FNS data, 13 experienced a decrease in SNAP E&T participation—ranging from a 21 percent decrease to a 93 percent decrease.[23] Overall, voluntary programs are generally smaller than mandatory programs, according to our analysis of FNS data.[24] In fiscal year 2016, for example, the 32 states or territories operating voluntary programs together served less than half of the total number of SNAP E&T participants served by the 21 states or territories operating mandatory programs, although these two groups of states had similar numbers of new work registrants.[25] Furthermore, states operating voluntary programs served an average of nearly 7,000 SNAP E&T

---

[23] Over the same period, 9 of the 13 states or territories that changed from a mandatory to a voluntary program and experienced a decrease in SNAP E&T participation experienced an increase in their total number of SNAP work registrants. In the 9 additional states or territories that changed from a mandatory to a voluntary programs and experienced an increase in SNAP E&T participation, this increase ranged from 3 percent to 954 percent. In the latter case, participation in one state increased from 13 participants in fiscal year 2010 to 137 in fiscal year 2011.

[24] Program size may be affected by multiple factors. Although SNAP recipients choose whether or not to participate in voluntary programs, in mandatory programs, some work registrants may fail to participate while others may be exempted from participation. For example, state SNAP agencies may elect to exempt from participation in mandatory E&T programs categories and individuals for whom participation is judged impractical or not cost effective. According to agency guidance, exemptions may be based on categories of individuals, such as those who live in certain areas; characteristics of individuals, such as those with low literacy; or significant access barriers, such as a lack of transportation, dependent care, or computer access.

[25] In fiscal year 2016, the 32 states operating voluntary programs had a combined 2.9 million new work registrants and the 21 states operating mandatory programs had a combined 3.2 million new work registrants.

participants per state, while states operating mandatory programs served an average of 23,000 SNAP E&T participants per state.

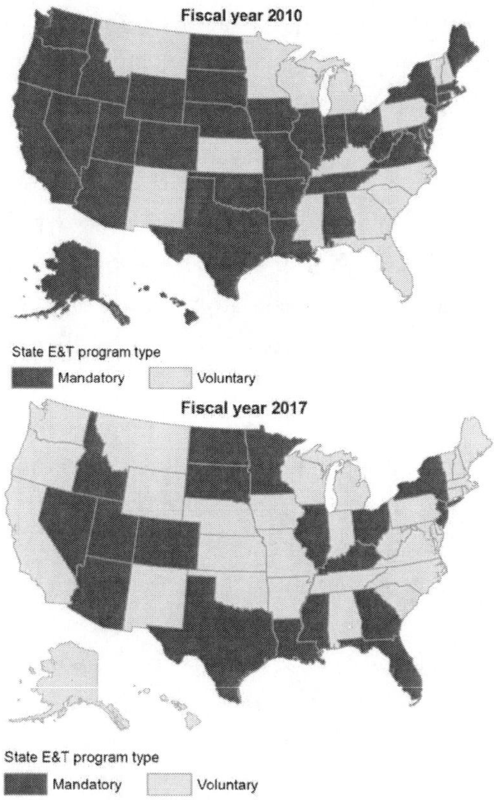

Source: GAO analysis of Food and Nutrition Service (FNS) Supplemental Nutrition Assistance Program (SNAP) E7T program data. | GAO-18-504T.

Note: Some states operate mandatory SNAP E&T programs in certain localities rather than statewide. These states are denoted as having mandatory programs in the figure. Guam and the Virgin Islands are not included in the figure. In fiscal year 2010, Guam operated a voluntary program. In fiscal year 2017, Guam, the District of Columbia, and the Virgin Islands operated voluntary programs.

Figure 3. SNAP Employment and Training (E&T) Program Type, Fiscal Years 2010 and 2017.

Focus on ABAWDs Has Increased as Waivers Have Expired

Evidence suggests that states have increased their focus on serving ABAWDs—a sub-population of SNAP recipients subject to benefit time limits and additional work requirements—through SNAP E&T, as related waivers have expired in recent years, according to FNS data. During and after the 2007-2009 recession, the majority of states operated under statewide waivers of the ABAWD time limit due to economic conditions. However, as the economy recovered, most statewide waivers expired, and the ABAWD time limit was reinstated. For example, according to FNS data, in fiscal year 2011, 45 states or territories had a statewide waiver and 7 states had a partial waiver—one applying to certain localities. By fiscal year 2017, the number of states or territories with a statewide waiver had decreased to 9, while 27 states had partial waivers.[26] FNS officials and state SNAP agency officials we spoke with in some states told us that, as the waivers have ended, state SNAP E&T programs have become increasingly focused on serving ABAWDs.[27]

Although state data on SNAP E&T programs reported to FNS suggest a greater percentage of ABAWDs have been participating in these programs in recent years, according to FNS officials, these data have limited usefulness in assessing state trends in serving ABAWDs for several reasons. For example, in recent years, FNS officials learned that there was widespread confusion among states regarding the need to track ABAWDs when waivers were in place, and that as a result, some states had not been tracking ABAWDs or properly documenting SNAP recipients' ABAWD status.[28] This is consistent with what some of the selected states we spoke

---

[26] The 9 states or territories with statewide waivers in fiscal year 2017 were Alaska, California, District of Columbia, Guam, Illinois, Louisiana, Nevada, New Mexico, and the Virgin Islands.

[27] According to FNS data, as waivers have expired in recent years, some states have also made use of additional exemptions to extend SNAP eligibility beyond 3 months for ABAWDs subject to the time limit for up to 15 percent of a state's ABAWDs subject to the time limits. Specifically, in fiscal year 2016, 33 states and territories made use of the 15 percent exemptions.

[28] FNS officials told us that states should have continued to track ABAWDs even if the state was under a statewide ABAWD waiver. Furthermore, in a memorandum to regional directors, FNS noted the importance of accurately tracking ABAWDs following the expiration of the waivers and reinstatement of the time limit, writing that states that failed to do so risked potential overpayments and Quality Control errors. Specifically, an ABAWD who fails to

with reported. As part of our ongoing work, we are continuing to explore the availability and reliability of data on ABAWDs.

States Increasingly Developed Partnerships to Deliver SNAP E&T Services

State SNAP agencies have increasingly partnered with other state and local organizations, such as workforce agencies, community-based social service providers, and community colleges, to provide services to SNAP E&T participants in recent years, according to FNS and states we selected for our review. In fiscal year 2018, nearly all states partnered with at least one other organization to deliver SNAP E&T services, with the majority partnering with more than one, according to an analysis by FNS.[29]

In recent years, FNS has urged states to make use of the broad network of American Job Centers. The American Job Centers, also known as one-stop centers, are funded through the Department of Labor's Employment and Training Administration and designed to provide a range of employment-related services, such as training referrals, career counseling, job listings, and similar employment-related services, to job seekers under one roof.[30] Our prior work has highlighted the value of coordination between federally funded employment and training programs to ensure the efficient and effective use of resources.[31] Despite encouraging such partnerships, FNS officials said that American Job Centers typically provide lighter touch services to SNAP E&T participants, such as job search and job search training, and they therefore may not be well suited for SNAP E&T participants who have multiple barriers to employment. In

comply with the SNAP work requirement within the time period is no longer eligible for SNAP; if the non-compliant ABAWD is not properly identified, this could lead to an overpayment.

[29] Kansas, New Hampshire, and New Mexico administer SNAP E&T programs that are solely operated by their state SNAP agencies.

[30] The American Job Centers were established under the Workforce Investment Act of 1998 and reauthorized in the Workforce Innovation and Opportunity Act. The Workforce Innovation and Opportunity Act aims, in part, to increase coordination among federal workforce development programs.

[31] GAO, *Multiple Employment and Training Programs: Providing Information on Colocating Services and Consolidating Administrative Structures Could Promote Efficiencies,* GAO-11-92 (Washington, D.C.: January 13, 2011).

our 2003 work on SNAP E&T, we found that while workforce system programs offered some of the activities needed by SNAP E&T participants, officials from 12 of the 15 states we contacted said that most participants were not ready for these activities, in part, because they lacked basic skills, such as reading and computer literacy, that would allow them to successfully participate.[32]

An alternative service delivery strategy that FNS has promoted is the development of third party partnerships with community-based social service providers, community colleges, and other entities to help states enhance their SNAP E&T programs. According to FNS, in this model, third party organizations use non-federal funding to provide allowable SNAP E&T services and supports, which are then eligible for 50 percent federal reimbursement funds through the state's SNAP E&T program.[33] According to FNS officials, third party partnerships enable states to leverage additional resources, grow their SNAP E&T programs, and reach more SNAP participants. In addition, FNS officials said that these partnerships allow states to improve their program outcomes by tapping into providers currently serving communities that include SNAP recipients. Federal 50 percent reimbursement funds expended increased from nearly $182 million to more than $223 million, or by 23 percent, from fiscal year 2007 to fiscal year 2016.[34]

---

[32] Officials from 5 of those states said that mental health problems often prevented SNAP E&T participants from participating in more intensive employment and training programs at one-stops. GAO-03-388. A 2017 FNS study that surveyed SNAP E&T participants about their barriers to obtaining or retaining employment found that while 20 percent of respondents reported no barriers, 28 percent reported one barrier, and 52 percent reported two or more barriers. The most frequently reported barriers were transportation issues, physical or mental health issues, lack of education, and having a criminal record. Rowe, Gretchen, Elizabeth Brown, and Brian Estes. *SNAP Employment and Training (E&T) Characteristics Study: Final Report.* Prepared by Mathematica Policy Research for the U.S. Department of Agriculture, Food and Nutrition Service, October 2017.

[33] These funding sources can include state training funds for specific populations, county and city funds, foundation or corporate funds, and social enterprise funds, according to FNS.

[34] States receive 50 percent reimbursement funds from the federal government for (1) administrative costs beyond the amount funded through 100 percent funds (described below), and (2) payments made by the states to participants for expenses reasonably related to participation in the program, like transportation and dependent care. According to FNS, states are required to reimburse participants for expenses that are necessary for participation in SNAP E&T.

FNS Has Taken Steps to Increase Support and Oversight of SNAP E&T

FNS has taken steps to increase federal support of states' SNAP E&T programs by increasing the number of federal staff responsible for SNAP E&T and providing additional technical assistance to states. Specifically, FNS officials said that in 2014, they created the Office of Employment and Training to provide support and oversight for the SNAP E&T program and expanded SNAP E&T staff in FNS headquarters from one to five fulltime employees. FNS has also taken steps to increase technical assistance to states. For example, they have developed tools, including the SNAP E&T Operations Handbook, intended to help states implement and grow their program, and by adding a dedicated SNAP E&T official in each of FNS's seven regional offices. According to FNS, regional officials have targeted technical assistance to states on, for example, developing third-party partnerships, and they have emphasized evidence-based approaches to administering the program, such as providing skills-based training for in-demand occupations.

FNS officials rely on various information sources to oversee states' SNAP E&T programs, including participant outcome data reported by states for the first time in January 2018. For example, FNS officials conduct management evaluation reviews of states, annually review states' SNAP E&T plans for compliance, and collect data from states on program participation and expenditures. In addition, as of January 2018, FNS has begun receiving new data on SNAP E&T program participants and outcomes from states.[35] These data include employment outcomes, such as the number of SNAP E&T participants in unsubsidized employment after participation in the program, and participant characteristics, such as the number of participants entering the program with a high school degree or

[35] The Agriculture Act of 2014 required that USDA, in consultation with the Department of Labor, develop reporting measures and that USDA require states to report outcome data to USDA on an annual basis. That Act also specified that the measures be based on common measures of performance for federal workforce training programs. Pub. L. No. 113-79, § 4022(a)(2), 128 Stat. 649, 805. FNS issued an interim rule implementing the reporting measures in March 2016. 81 Fed. Reg. 15,613 (Mar. 24, 2016).

equivalent. FNS officials said that although states generally submitted the new data on time, states experienced challenges that likely affected the accuracy of the data. For example, some states needed to manually collect data on participant characteristics due to the limited capacity of their data systems. Further, according to FNS officials, some states did not correctly interpret certain reporting definitions or time periods. To address these challenges, FNS officials have been providing technical assistance to states to help them refine their participant and outcome data reports. Officials told us that they expect the states to submit revised reports by May 2018; we will examine these data and related issues in our ongoing work.

FNS Has Taken Steps to Address SNAP Program Integrity Issues, but Concerns Remain

FNS and the states partner to address issues that affect program integrity, including improper payments and fraud, and FNS has taken some steps to address challenges in these areas, but concerns remain. For example, regarding SNAP recipient and retailer fraud, FNS has taken some steps to address challenges identified in our 2006 and 2014 reports related to fraud committed by SNAP recipients and authorized retailers, but more remains to be done. We currently have ongoing work to assess the steps FNS and states have taken to address our recommendations related to recipient and retailer fraud and other program vulnerabilities.

SNAP Improper Payments

In 2016, we reviewed SNAP improper payment rates and found that states' adoption of program flexibilities and changes in federal SNAP policy in the previous decade, as well as improper payment rate calculation methods, likely affected these rates.[36] For example, when states adopted

[36] GAO-16-708T.

available SNAP policy flexibilities that simplified or lessened participant reporting requirements, these changes reduced the opportunity for error and led to a decline in the improper payment rate, according to a USDA study. In addition, we found that the methodology SNAP used to calculate its improper payment rate was generally similar to the methodologies used for other large federal programs for low-income individuals, including Medicaid, Earned Income Tax Credit, and Supplemental Security Income. However, we also found that some of the procedural and methodological differences in the rate calculation among these programs likely affected the resulting improper payment rates, such as how cases with insufficient information or certain kinds of errors were factored into the improper payment rate.[37]

In 2014, USDA identified SNAP improper payment data quality issues in some states and has since been working with the states to improve improper payment estimates. Although USDA reported national SNAP improper payment estimates for benefits paid through fiscal year 2014, USDA did not report a national SNAP improper payment estimate for benefits paid in fiscal years 2015 or 2016.[38] In response to a report from USDA's Office of Inspector General that identified concerns in the application of SNAP's quality control process, which is used to identify improper payments, USDA began a review of state quality control systems in all states in 2014.[39] According to USDA, due to the data quality issues uncovered in 42 of 53 states during the reviews, the improper payment

[37] For example, SNAP excludes certain errors from its improper payment calculation. Specifically, SNAP excludes errors below a specific dollar threshold from its improper payment rate calculation, and FNS's data on payment errors suggests that the threshold has a direct effect on the SNAP improper payment rate. According to federal officials, the other federal programs for low-income individuals we reviewed did not exclude errors below a specific dollar threshold.

[38] USDA reports its estimate of SNAP benefits improperly paid in a specific fiscal year in the following year's agency financial report. As such, USDA did not report SNAP improper payment estimates in its fiscal year 2016 and 2017 agency financial reports.

[39] The OIG found that states weakened the quality control process by using third-party consultants and error review committees to mitigate individual quality control-identified errors, rather than improve eligibility determinations; and that quality control staff also treated error cases non-uniformly. The OIG concluded that FNS' quality control process may have understated SNAP's improper payment rate. USDA, Office of Inspector General, *FNS Quality Control Process for SNAP Error Rate*, September, 2015.

rates for those states could not be validated, and the department was unable to calculate a national improper payment rate for benefits paid in fiscal year 2015.[40] To address the data quality concerns, USDA updated guidance, provided training to relevant state and federal staff, and worked with states to update their procedures to ensure consistency with federal guidelines. According to USDA, the department also required individual states to develop corrective action plans to address issues identified and monitored progress to ensure states took identified actions. On June 30, 2017, USDA notified the states that the department would not release a national SNAP improper payment rate for benefits paid in fiscal year 2016 and remained focused on conducting the fiscal year 2017 review.

SNAP Recipient Fraud

FNS has increased its oversight of state anti-fraud activities in recent years by developing new guidance and providing training and technical assistance to states on detecting fraud by SNAP recipients and reporting on anti-fraud activities to FNS.[41] In 2014, we reported on 11 selected states' efforts to combat SNAP recipient fraud and made several recommendations to FNS to address the challenges states faced.[42] We found that FNS and states faced challenges in the following areas:

---

[40] USDA reviewed the quality control systems in the 50 states, District of Columbia, Guam, and the Virgin Islands. USDA released state error rates for the 11 states whose quality control data could be validated.

[41] Little is known about the extent of recipient fraud in the SNAP program nationwide beyond data from investigations. According to a September 2012 USDA OIG report, the magnitude of program abuse due to recipient fraud is unknown because states do not have uniform ways of compiling, tracking, and reporting their recipient fraud rates. The USDA OIG recommended that FNS determine the feasibility of creating a uniform methodology for states to calculate their recipient fraud rate. U.S. Department of Agriculture, Office of Inspector General, *Analysis of FNS' Supplemental Nutrition Assistance Program Fraud Prevention and Detection Efforts,* Audit Report 27002-001-13, September 2012, p. 2, https://www.usda.gov/oig/webdocs/27002-0011-13.pdf. In 2014, FNS responded to the OIG that it had determined that it would be infeasible to implement as it would require legislative authority mandating significant state investment of time and resources in investigating, prosecuting and reporting fraud beyond current requirements.

[42] GAO, *Supplemental Nutrition Assistance Program: Enhanced Detection Tools and Reporting Could Improve Efforts to Combat Recipient Fraud,* GAO-14-641 (Washington, D.C.: August 21, 2014).

- Guidance on use of data tools to detect fraud: States faced challenges using FNS-recommended data tools to detect fraud, and FNS is in the process of developing improved guidance to address this concern. Specifically, FNS's guidance on the use of EBT transaction data to uncover potential patterns of benefit trafficking lacked the specificity states needed to uncover such activity, and we recommended FNS develop additional guidance. Since then, FNS contracted with a private consulting firm to provide 10 states with technical assistance in recipient fraud prevention and detection, which included exploring the use of data analytics to analyze and interpret eligibility and transaction data to identify patterns or trends and create models that incorporate predictive analytics. FNS officials also recently told us that the agency is developing a SNAP Fraud Framework to provide guidance to states on improving fraud prevention and detection. FNS officials anticipated releasing the framework in mid- 2018.
- Tools for monitoring e-commerce websites: We also found FNS-recommended tools for automatically monitoring potential SNAP trafficking on e-commerce websites to be of limited use and less effective than manual searches, and FNS has developed but not finalized guidance on using such tools. We recommended that FNS reassess the effectiveness of its current guidance and tools for states to monitor e-commerce and social media websites. In August 2017, FNS officials told us that they had developed revised guidance for states on using social media in detection of SNAP trafficking. According to FNS, the guidance will be incorporated into the SNAP Fraud Framework.
- Staff levels: During the time of our 2014 work, most of our 11 selected states reported difficulties conducting fraud investigations due to reduced or stagnant staff levels while numbers of SNAP recipients had greatly increased, but FNS decided not to make changes to address this issue. Specifically, 8 of the 11 states we reviewed reported inadequate staffing due to attrition, turnover, or lack of funding. Some states suggested changing the financial

incentive structure to promote fraud investigations because agencies were not rewarded for cost-effective, anti-fraud efforts that could prevent ineligible people from receiving benefits. Specifically, when fraud by a SNAP recipient is discovered, a state may generally retain 35 percent of any recovered overpayments. However, there are no recovered funds when a state detects potential fraud by an applicant and denies the application. To help address states' concerns about resources needed to conduct investigations, we recommended in our 2014 report that FNS explore ways that federal financial incentives could be used to better support cost-effective anti-fraud strategies. FNS reported that it took some steps to explore alternative financial incentives, through a review of responses to a Request for Information in the Federal Register.[43] However, FNS decided not to pursue bonus awards for anti-fraud and program integrity activities. Given that FNS has not made changes in this area, state SNAP fraud agencies may continue to report resource concerns in addressing fraud.

- Reporting guidance: We also found that FNS did not have consistent and reliable data on states' activities because of unclear reporting guidance, and FNS has since revised its data collection form and provided training on the changes. To improve FNS's ability to monitor states and obtain information about more efficient and effective ways to combat recipient fraud, we recommended in 2014 that FNS take steps, such as providing guidance and training, to enhance the consistency of what states report on their anti-fraud activities. In response, FNS revised the form used to collect recipient integrity information and changed the reporting frequency from annual to quarterly, effective fiscal year 2017. FNS officials also reported providing training to

[43] According to FNS officials, FNS considered changes to its bonus structure, such as including a new category for high or most improved performance in recipient integrity. FNS also encouraged states to use funds from existing performance bonuses to improve program administration, particularly in the area of program integrity.

approximately 400 state agency and FNS regional office personnel on the updates to the form and related instructions.

In our ongoing work, we are further reviewing states' use of data analytics to identify SNAP recipient fraud, including that which may be occurring during out-of-state transactions. Because transactions that may appear suspicious—such as those made out-of-state—may in fact be legitimate, states may use data analytic techniques to include additional factors that may help them better target their efforts to identify potential fraud. However, states may have different levels of capacity for using data analytics to detect fraud. We are examining how 7 selected states are using data analytics and identifying the advantages and challenges states have experienced in doing so. We are also assessing FNS's efforts to assist states in implementing GAO's leading practices for data analytics outlined in GAO's Framework for Managing Fraud Risks in Federal Programs outlined in GAO's Framework for Managing Fraud Risks in Federal Programs.[44] In addition, we are conducting our own analysis of EBT out-of-state SNAP transaction data. We expect to report on our findings later this year.

SNAP Retailer Trafficking

FNS has taken some steps to prevent, detect, and respond to retailers who traffic SNAP benefits since our last report on the issue in 2006,[45] but trafficking continues to be a problem. For example, in February 2018, a federal jury convicted a grocery store operator in Baltimore on charges of wire fraud in connection with a scheme to traffic more than $1.6 million in

---

[44] GAO, *A Framework for Managing Fraud Risks in Federal Programs*, GAO-15-593SP (Washington, D.C.: July 2015).

[45] GAO, *Food Stamp Trafficking: FNS Could Enhance Program Integrity by Better Targeting Stores Likely to Traffic and Increasing Penalties.* GAO-07-53. (Washington, D.C.: Oct. 13, 2006).

SNAP benefits for food sales that never occurred.[46] The grocery store operator paid cash for SNAP benefits, typically paying the recipient half the value of the benefits and keeping the other half for himself. In our 2006 report, we found that SNAP was vulnerable to retailer trafficking in several areas, including:

- Requirements for food that retailers must stock to participate in SNAP: In 2006, we found that FNS had minimal requirements for the amounts of food that retailers must stock, which could allow retailers more likely to traffic into the program, although the agency has since taken steps to increase these requirements. In our 2006 report, FNS officials said that they authorized stores with limited food stock to provide access to food in low-income areas where large grocery stores were scarce. At that time, retailers were generally required to stock a minimum of 12 food items (at least 3 varieties of 4 staple food categories, such as fruits and vegetables), but FNS rules did not specify how many items of each variety would constitute sufficient stock.[47] FNS officials told us that a retailer that only carries small quantities of food, such as a few cans of one kind of vegetable, may intend to traffic. In 2016, FNS promulgated a final rule increasing food stock requirements.[48] FNS officials told us that these new rules are designed to encourage stores to provide more healthy food options for recipients and discourage trafficking. According to FNS, retailers are now generally required to stock at least 36 food items (a certain variety and quantity of staple foods in each of the 4 staple food categories).[49]

---

[46] Department of Justice, "Catonsville Man Convicted for Food Stamp Fraud." (Baltimore, MD: Feb. 20, 2018).

[47] Alternatively, retailers could meet a second criterion for authorization, which required the store to have more than 50 percent of its sales in a staple food group, such as meat, poultry, or fish.

[48] 81 Fed. Reg. 90,675 (Dec. 15, 2016).

[49] Retailers can still meet the second criterion that more than 50 percent of its sales are in a staple food group. Stores that do not meet either criterion may still be considered for authorization

- Focus on high-risk retailers: We also found in 2006 that FNS had not conducted analyses to identify characteristics of retailers at high risk of trafficking and to target its resources—a shortcoming FNS has since taken some steps to address. For example, we reported that some stores may be at risk of trafficking because one or more previous owners had been found trafficking at the same location. However, FNS did not have a system in place to ensure that these retailers were quickly targeted for heightened attention. In addition, once a store was authorized to participate in the program, FNS staff typically would not inspect the store again until it applied for reauthorization 5 years later.[50] We recommended that FNS identify the stores most likely to traffic and provide earlier, more targeted oversight to those stores. In 2009, FNS began establishing risk levels for each authorized retailer, identifying high-risk stores as those with a prior permanent disqualification at that location or a nearby location.[51] In 2013, FNS required all high-risk retailers to go through reauthorization and to provide additional documentation regarding store ownership.[52] That same year, FNS also consolidated its retailer management functions, including those for authorizing stores and analyzing EBT transaction data, into a single national structure known as the Retailer Operations Division. FNS officials told us that this structure enables the agency to identify and deploy their investigative resources to the areas of highest risk nationally, rather than within a given region.
- Penalties to deter retailer trafficking: We also found in our 2006 report that FNS's penalties for retailer trafficking may be

---

if they are located in an area where SNAP recipients have significantly limited access to food.

[50] After a retailer applies for authorization, an FNS contractor conducts an on-site inspection at the store to verify information from the application and take pictures of the store and its inventory, including the condition of its food stock.

[51] Medium-risk stores, for example, include those with temporary disqualifications or other program violations, according to FNS.

[52] As part of our ongoing work, we will review FNS's current authorization and reauthorization processes for stores.

insufficient to deter traffickers, and since then, FNS has proposed—but not finalized—rules to increase them. FNS imposes administrative penalties for retailer trafficking—generally a permanent disqualification from the program or a monetary penalty.[53] FNS relies on the USDA Office of Inspector General (OIG) and other law enforcement entities to conduct investigations that can lead to criminal prosecutions.[54] In our 2006 report, we recommended that FNS develop a strategy to increase penalties for trafficking. The Food, Conservation, and Energy Act of 2008 (known as the 2008 Farm Bill) gave USDA authority to impose higher monetary penalties, and the authority to impose both a monetary penalty and program disqualification on retailers found to have violated relevant law or regulations (which includes those found to have trafficked).[55] In 2012, FNS proposed regulatory changes to implement these authorities. However, FNS has not finalized these rules, and as of fall 2017, the rules were considered "inactive."[56]

In our ongoing work, we are continuing to assess FNS's efforts to prevent, detect, and respond to retailer trafficking, as well as examining what is known about the extent of retailer trafficking nationwide. As part

---

[53] In lieu of program disqualification, FNS can assess a civil monetary penalty if a store demonstrates that it had an effective policy and program in effect to prevent violations of relevant law and regulations. In addition, FNS imposes a "transfer of ownership" penalty if the disqualified owner sells his or her store before the expiration of the disqualification period (and in the case of permanent disqualification, the penalty is double that for a ten year disqualification period).

[54] Specifically, the USDA OIG, U.S. Secret Service, and Federal Bureau of Investigation conduct investigations that can lead to criminal prosecutions. However, in 2006, we found that these entities were conducting fewer of these resource-intensive investigations, instead focusing on high-impact investigations. According to the USDA OIG, it opened fewer trafficking investigations because it had fewer investigators and decided to focus its resources on high-impact cases, such as those with large-scale trafficking or involving other criminal activity.

[55] Specifically, the 2008 Farm Bill gave FNS the authority to increase penalties to up to $100,000 for each violation. Pub. L. No. 110-246, § 4132, 122 Stat. 1651, 1875.

[56] The Office of Information and Regulatory Affairs publishes the "Inactive List" of regulatory actions under agency review but not included on the "Unified Agenda" of rules planned to be implemented in the near or future term. Agencies designate actions as "inactive" when they choose to take additional time to review a regulatory or deregulatory action but wish to preserve the regulatory identification number and title for possible future use.

of this work, we are continuing to review FNS's response to our prior recommendations, as well as related recommendations made by USDA's OIG.[57] We are also studying FNS's periodic estimates of the rate of retailer trafficking, expressed as the dollar value and percentage of all SNAP benefits that were trafficked and the percentage of retailers involved. These data suggest an increase in the estimated rate of retailer trafficking since our 2006 report. However, we and others, including a group of experts convened by FNS, have identified some limitations with the retailer trafficking estimates.[58] For example, the trafficking rate is calculated based on a sample of retailers that FNS considers most likely to traffic. Although FNS adjusts the data to better represent the broader population of authorized retailers, it is uncertain whether the resulting estimates accurately reflect the extent of trafficking nationwide. We are reviewing these limitations and FNS's efforts to address them in our ongoing work.

Chairman Jordan, Chairman Palmer, Ranking Member Krishnamoorthi, Ranking Member Raskin, and Members of the Subcommittees, this completes my prepared statement. I would be pleased to respond to any questions that you may have at this time.

---

[57] See, for example, USDA Office of Inspector General, *FNS: Controls for Authorizing Supplemental Nutrition Assistance Program Retailers.* Audit Report 27601-0001-31 (Washington, D.C.: July 2013).

[58] See USDA Office of Inspector General, *Analysis of FNS' Supplemental Nutrition Assistance Program Fraud Prevention and Detection Efforts.* Audit Report 27002-0011-13 (Washington, D.C.: September 2012). In addition, in 2013, FNS convened a technical working group of outside experts to assess its trafficking estimates methodology and propose alternatives.

INDEX

A

access, xi, 4, 14, 17, 22, 40, 57, 82, 100, 111, 112, 120, 121, 129, 131, 133, 136, 145, 153, 155, 162, 163, 187, 233, 245, 246
adults, 34, 37, 49, 67, 68, 71, 98, 112, 127, 135, 212, 219, 224, 228, 229
advocacy, 5, 7, 22, 25, 123, 128
after school, x, 39, 49, 80
age, xiii, 11, 12, 37, 38, 46, 49, 50, 67, 70, 73, 95, 112, 113, 124, 125, 126, 145, 151, 166, 174, 178, 181, 203, 207, 208, 220, 224, 231
agencies, xii, xiii, xiv, 15, 30, 44, 52, 57, 75, 81, 82, 83, 90, 94, 97, 103, 106, 107, 114, 116, 123, 128, 130, 132, 133, 134, 135, 136, 137, 142, 144, 145, 146, 147, 152, 154, 157, 163, 166, 167, 169, 173, 175, 176, 179, 180, 181, 184, 185, 186, 187, 188, 189, 190, 191, 192, 193, 196, 198, 200, 204, 206, 207, 208, 210, 211, 212, 213, 221, 224, 225, 227, 232, 233, 236, 243
agricultural producers, 13
agriculture, 41, 44, 82, 97
appropriations, ix, x, xi, xii, 2, 4, 8, 11, 18, 19, 26, 33, 35, 36, 38, 40, 45, 48, 70, 77, 79, 82, 83, 100, 111, 120, 153, 170, 171, 182, 192, 197, 200
awareness, 92, 105, 122, 123, 128, 147, 159

B

benefits, viii, xiii, xiv, 17, 38, 42, 44, 56, 77, 98, 108, 111, 112, 154, 166, 167, 169, 170, 173, 178, 179, 180, 181, 182, 183, 184, 186, 187, 189, 190, 191, 193, 204, 208, 217, 219, 220, 221, 223, 224, 226, 227, 240, 243, 244, 248
breastfeeding, xii, xiii, xiv, 38, 70, 112, 165, 166, 167, 172, 173, 179, 180, 181, 183, 184, 185, 196, 199, 203, 204, 208
Buy American, ix, 2, 14, 15, 16

C

cash, xi, xiii, 40, 41, 47, 50, 56, 64, 65, 68, 73, 74, 75, 96, 166, 169, 182, 187, 191, 196, 198, 199, 220, 221, 227, 245

Census, xii, 90, 97, 117, 118, 121, 142, 144, 148, 149, 150, 152, 154
certification, xi, 8, 22, 40, 53, 56, 57, 59, 71, 82, 172, 177, 179, 185, 195
challenges, vii, xii, 7, 90, 91, 93, 116, 117, 119, 122, 123, 125, 129, 131, 133, 134, 135, 136, 138, 142, 143, 144, 145, 146, 147, 154, 155, 160, 163, 191, 219, 221, 239, 241, 242, 244
cheese, 26, 181
Child and Adult Care Food Pro, vii, viii, x, 1, 3, 5, 31, 34, 39, 41, 43, 49, 67, 69, 70, 74, 80, 84, 87, 89, 112, 139
child nutrition, v, vii, viii, x, xiii, 1, 3, 4, 5, 6, 8, 11, 12, 14, 15, 17, 19, 21, 22, 28, 30, 33, 34, 35, 37, 38, 39, 40, 41, 42, 43, 44, 45, 46, 47, 48, 49, 50, 53, 55, 57, 62, 67, 70, 74, 76, 77, 78, 79, 80, 81, 82, 83, 84, 85, 93, 97, 98, 99, 103, 107, 109, 121, 131, 133, 135, 136, 138, 139, 142, 152, 155, 156, 158, 161, 163, 165, 167, 168, 172, 178, 182, 188, 191, 204
Child Nutrition Act, x, xiii, 4, 5, 33, 37, 38, 41, 43, 49, 50, 53, 82, 99, 165, 167, 168, 172, 178, 204
child nutrition programs, v, vii, viii, x, xiii, 1, 3, 4, 5, 8, 11, 17, 19, 21, 28, 33, 34, 35, 39, 40, 41, 42, 43, 45, 46, 47, 48, 49, 55, 62, 67, 70, 77, 78, 80, 81, 82, 84, 93, 97, 98, 107, 121, 133, 135, 136, 138, 142, 152, 155, 163, 165, 168
child poverty, xii, 90, 154
childhood, xi, 37, 40, 49, 67
commodity, xi, 34, 40, 41, 43, 47, 50, 64, 66, 67, 68, 69, 70, 73, 74, 75, 81, 86, 87
community, xi, 22, 23, 36, 37, 40, 47, 49, 60, 65, 75, 81, 95, 97, 98, 105, 114, 119, 122, 123, 125, 126, 129, 134, 144, 236, 237
Community Eligibility Provision (CEP), ix, 2, 4, 21, 22, 23, 31, 54, 59, 60, 64, 66, 84
Congress, viii, ix, x, xii, 1, 2, 3, 4, 5, 8, 11, 12, 13, 15, 16, 18, 19, 21, 22, 23, 24, 25, 26, 28, 30, 33, 40, 43, 44, 45, 59, 62, 77, 80, 93, 99, 100, 120, 122, 132, 137, 153, 162, 168, 171, 179, 182, 197
Consolidated Appropriations Act, 100, 107, 111, 130, 133, 153, 158, 162
consumption, 4, 13, 17, 18, 21, 42, 82, 145, 197, 205, 212
consumption habits, 145
cost, viii, 16, 23, 28, 48, 53, 75, 76, 88, 99, 115, 117, 119, 153, 167, 173, 186, 187, 188, 190, 191, 192, 196, 200, 221, 233, 243

D

data collection, 145, 198, 243
database, 59, 170, 172
day care, x, 37, 39, 41, 43, 44, 46, 49, 67, 68, 69, 70, 71, 72, 73, 74, 87, 112, 135
demographic characteristics, 193, 231
demonstrations, 20, 100, 111, 120, 122, 153
Department of Agriculture, 196, 197, 207
Department of Defense, 139, 140, 169
Department of Health and Human Services, 98, 209
Department of Justice, 245
Department of Labor, 236, 238
diet, 178, 180, 209, 220
Dietary Guidelines, 6, 61, 82, 197, 199, 209
Dietary Guidelines for Americans, 6, 61, 82, 197, 199, 209
disability, 95, 152, 228, 229
distribution, xiv, 25, 47, 64, 81, 138, 167, 184
drug abuse, xiv, 166, 178, 184

E

education, xii, xiv, 23, 24, 44, 52, 82, 83, 112, 127, 165, 166, 167, 172, 180, 184, 185, 203, 208, 225, 226, 237
educational materials, 185
elementary school, xi, 3, 26, 38, 40, 50, 74
eligibility, vii, viii, ix, xi, xiii, 2, 22, 23, 31, 36, 37, 40, 42, 45, 47, 49, 53, 54, 55, 57, 59, 60, 68, 71, 73, 74, 75, 76, 78, 80, 81, 98, 118, 120, 121, 129, 134, 142, 146, 148, 149, 150, 152, 166, 167, 173, 174, 175, 176, 177, 178, 179, 185, 198, 205, 220, 221, 223, 224, 225, 226, 227, 235, 240, 242
eligibility criteria, xi, 40, 45, 53, 73, 80
employment, 218, 221, 224, 225, 227, 232, 236, 237, 238
expenditures, xii, xiv, 38, 45, 70, 78, 83, 90, 93, 96, 218, 221, 225, 238

F

families, 26, 48, 54, 60, 71, 72, 97, 99, 109, 114, 121, 123, 126, 147, 175
family income, 54, 72, 75, 79, 175, 185
family members, 169
farmers, 16, 34, 38, 82, 200
fat, 6, 9, 10, 11, 61, 62, 70, 197
federal aid, 46, 68
federal assistance, 68, 72
Federal Bureau of Investigation, 228, 247
federal funds, xiii, 15, 24, 28, 67, 166, 171, 172
federal government, xi, 3, 28, 40, 44, 99, 153, 170, 204, 206, 221, 226, 227, 237
federal law, xi, xii, xiv, 40, 57, 90, 94, 134, 139, 154, 167, 190, 191, 204, 206, 220, 222, 224
Federal Register, 3, 6, 8, 11, 25, 26, 28, 30, 55, 59, 60, 61, 62, 64, 70, 74, 83, 84, 85, 86, 87, 176, 196, 197, 243
federal regulations, 24, 55, 169, 171
federal workforce, 236, 238
financial, xiii, 24, 26, 30, 41, 45, 53, 73, 75, 117, 166, 173, 226, 240, 242
financial incentives, 243
financial reports, 240
financial support, 41, 53
fiscal year, xii, xiv, 64, 65, 66, 74, 79, 82, 90, 91, 92, 93, 96, 100, 101, 102, 103, 104, 112, 118, 121, 128, 129, 133, 136, 139, 140, 142, 143, 148, 149, 150, 151, 153, 154, 155, 156, 157, 162, 171, 204, 208, 217, 218, 219, 220, 221, 225, 226, 227, 228, 229, 232, 233, 234, 235, 236, 237, 240, 243
flexibility, 30, 49, 74, 92, 121, 130, 131, 132, 133, 137, 155, 160, 161, 162, 169, 175, 196, 219, 225, 232
food, vii, viii, x, xi, xii, xiii, xiv, 1, 3, 4, 7, 8, 12, 15, 16, 17, 18, 20, 23, 24, 26, 28, 29, 30, 31, 34, 36, 37, 39, 40, 41, 42, 43, 47, 49, 52, 54, 64, 65, 66, 67, 68, 69, 70, 75, 76, 77, 81, 83, 85, 86, 90, 92, 100, 107, 108, 109, 110, 111, 112, 113, 114, 115, 120, 122, 123, 124, 125, 133, 135, 142, 145, 151, 153, 162, 166, 168, 169, 170, 172, 173, 178, 180, 181, 182, 183, 184, 186, 187, 188, 189, 190, 191, 192, 193, 195, 196, 197, 198, 199, 200, 204, 205, 207, 208, 209, 212, 220, 221, 223, 227, 245, 246
Food and Drug Administration, 100, 111, 120, 130, 133, 153, 162, 214, 215
food industry, 5
food intake, 18, 112, 197, 204
food safety, 16, 36, 83
food security, 18, 112, 120, 122

formula, xiii, 27, 28, 30, 42, 46, 60, 79, 81, 82, 128, 166, 173, 181, 185, 188, 189, 199, 207, 208, 225
fraud, viii, xiv, 217, 218, 219, 221, 226, 227, 239, 241, 242, 243, 244
Fresh Fruit and Vegetable Program (FFVP), vii, viii, ix, xi, 1, 2, 3, 5, 12, 13, 31, 35, 38, 40, 41, 43, 48, 50, 69, 79, 80, 84
fruits, ix, xiii, 2, 6, 7, 13, 15, 16, 18, 61, 70, 80, 98, 166, 181, 191, 196, 199, 204, 205, 207, 208, 245
funding, vii, viii, ix, x, xi, xii, xiii, 2, 3, 4, 6, 17, 18, 19, 20, 23, 24, 28, 33, 35, 36, 37, 38, 40, 41, 42, 45, 47, 48, 49, 50, 51, 53, 54, 55, 60, 61, 63, 65, 66, 68, 69, 70, 77, 79, 81, 82, 83, 87, 97, 101, 112, 119, 120, 122, 126, 127, 128, 129, 133, 146, 152, 163, 166, 167, 170, 171, 172, 173, 179, 180, 192, 193, 200, 205, 225, 226, 233, 237, 242
funds, xi, xiii, 15, 24, 26, 28, 35, 36, 40, 45, 47, 64, 72, 74, 79, 97, 107, 111, 123, 128, 152, 166, 169, 170, 171, 172, 179, 186, 200, 201, 225, 226, 237, 243

G

governments, 123
grant programs, 34
grants, 18, 19, 35, 57, 79, 81, 82, 119, 127, 137, 160, 169, 172, 180, 181, 200, 204, 225, 226
guidance, xii, 5, 11, 12, 14, 15, 25, 30, 55, 90, 94, 96, 125, 131, 135, 136, 138, 139, 145, 152, 154, 161, 163, 187, 193, 198, 206, 210, 211, 212, 213, 219, 222, 227, 233, 241, 242, 243
guidelines, xi, 40, 46, 47, 54, 55, 62, 63, 70, 72, 85, 97, 109, 152, 172, 174, 175, 176, 184, 186, 209, 241

H

health, xii, xiii, 8, 44, 71, 75, 76, 96, 97, 112, 135, 165, 166, 167, 169, 178, 181, 184, 185, 203, 204, 207, 208, 212, 237
health care, xii, 112, 165, 167, 207
health care professionals, 207
health condition, 178
health problems, 167
health services, xiii, 166
health status, 167, 184
Healthy, Hunger-Free Kids Act of 2010 (HHFKA), viii, ix, x, xi, xiii, 1, 2, 3, 4, 5, 6, 8, 21, 24, 27, 28, 29, 30, 31, 33, 36, 40, 43, 51, 56, 57, 59, 60, 61, 62, 63, 70, 74, 81, 82, 83, 84, 165, 168, 182, 186, 200
high school, 6, 7, 9, 26, 63, 66, 74, 238
high school degree, 238
higher education, 220, 224
House of Representatives, xii, 92, 99, 100, 132, 151, 153, 162, 214, 215, 217
household income, 53, 54, 72, 73, 76, 80, 183, 226, 227

I

income, vii, ix, xi, xii, xiii, 2, 34, 40, 42, 47, 51, 53, 54, 55, 56, 59, 71, 72, 73, 74, 78, 79, 80, 90, 91, 92, 93, 95, 97, 100, 108, 111, 112, 113, 120, 122, 134, 136, 138, 143, 144, 145, 147, 151, 153, 154, 159, 165, 166, 167, 171, 174, 175, 176, 177, 185, 200, 203, 208, 209, 220, 227, 240, 245
individuals, 42, 95, 97, 113, 151, 173, 175, 185, 206, 207, 210, 211, 212, 220, 221, 225, 227, 233, 240
infants, xii, xiii, 34, 38, 51, 70, 112, 165, 166, 167, 171, 174, 179, 180, 181, 185, 193, 196, 203, 204, 207, 208

inflation, 29, 47, 64, 72, 79, 84, 85, 98, 171, 183
information sharing, 119, 126, 128, 138, 160
insecurity, 20, 77, 100, 120, 153
institutional settings, vii, viii, x, 1, 3, 39, 40, 42, 48, 168
institutions, 34, 41, 44, 51, 63, 67, 68, 72, 74, 75, 78, 112, 129, 135
integrity, viii, xiv, 134, 187, 191, 192, 206, 217, 218, 219, 221, 239, 243
issues, vii, viii, ix, xiv, 2, 4, 5, 7, 23, 27, 43, 83, 92, 93, 107, 116, 119, 128, 129, 133, 137, 158, 159, 160, 192, 193, 217, 219, 237, 239, 240

J

jurisdiction, x, 4, 34, 43, 83, 168

L

law enforcement, 130, 247
laws, ix, xi, xii, 2, 4, 8, 14, 19, 35, 36, 40, 43, 45, 70, 79, 81, 85, 170, 171, 192
legislation, 4, 14, 24, 27, 35
legislative authority, 241
legislative proposals, 5, 30
low-income children, vii, xii, 23, 51, 53, 59, 71, 73, 79, 90, 91, 93, 100, 108, 111, 112, 113, 120, 122, 138, 144, 145, 147, 153, 154, 159
lunch shaming, ix, 2, 23, 24, 26, 27

M

majority, x, xi, xii, 22, 33, 40, 46, 63, 65, 68, 70, 80, 81, 92, 95, 101, 109, 114, 117, 122, 123, 136, 171, 177, 235, 236
management, 83, 96, 128, 133, 135, 163, 170, 186, 193, 238, 246
meal costs, ix, 2, 23, 24, 26, 27
meals and snacks, viii, x, 3, 37, 39, 40, 41, 46, 48, 49, 67, 68, 71, 76, 81
medical history, 178
metabolic disorders, 207
methodology, xv, 95, 138, 154, 218, 222, 240, 241, 248
military, 129, 139, 140, 175, 190

N

National Academy of Sciences, 61, 182
National Health and Nutrition Examination Survey (NHANES), 212
National Research Council, 196
National School Lunch Program, vii, viii, x, 1, 3, 5, 6, 8, 9, 14, 15, 16, 30, 31, 34, 39, 41, 42, 43, 44, 46, 49, 50, 59, 60, 62, 63, 64, 69, 80, 83, 84, 89, 93, 118, 139, 148, 149, 150, 154, 156
natural disaster, 95, 101, 156
nonprofit organizations, 75, 76, 93, 97, 152
nutrition, vii, viii, x, xi, xii, xiii, xiv, 1, 2, 3, 4, 5, 6, 7, 8, 9, 11, 12, 14, 19, 21, 22, 28, 30, 33, 34, 35, 36, 38, 39, 40, 41, 42, 43, 44, 45, 46, 47, 48, 51, 57, 61, 62, 63, 64, 67, 70, 71, 74, 76, 78, 79, 80, 81, 82, 83, 85, 90, 92, 93, 97, 98, 103, 107,108, 111, 112, 115, 120, 125, 133, 135, 136, 138, 139, 151, 152, 154, 155, 156, 158, 163, 165, 166, 167, 168, 172, 180, 181, 184, 185, 192, 193, 196, 203, 204, 205, 208, 217, 220
nutrition standards, viii, 1, 2, 5, 6, 8, 9, 11, 12, 36, 46, 51, 61, 62, 63, 70, 71, 103
nutritional assessment, 178
nutritional status, 18, 100, 120, 153, 212

O

officials, xii, xiv, 24, 25, 26, 90, 92, 93, 94, 101, 103, 104, 105, 106, 107, 108, 109, 110, 111, 113, 114, 115, 117, 119, 120, 121, 122, 123, 124, 125, 128, 129, 131, 132, 133, 134, 135, 136, 138, 139, 140, 141, 142, 143, 154, 155, 157, 158, 160, 161, 162, 163, 178, 206, 218, 222, 223, 226, 227, 229, 230, 231, 232, 233, 235, 236, 237, 238, 240, 242, 243, 245, 246
operating costs, 47, 97, 98, 115, 119, 152
operations, x, xii, 4, 20, 24, 33, 40, 83, 131, 169, 187
outreach, 92, 106, 107, 123, 128, 136, 143, 144, 145, 146, 154, 157, 159
oversight, viii, xiv, 81, 82, 133, 163, 166, 206, 218, 219, 221, 227, 238, 241, 246
ownership, 191, 246, 247

P

parents, 7, 13, 57, 123, 124, 129
participants, viii, xiii, xiv, 17, 18, 34, 38, 57, 71, 72, 73, 100, 111, 133, 153, 162, 166, 167, 169, 170, 172, 174, 175, 176, 177, 178, 179, 180, 182, 184, 185, 186, 187, 188, 189, 190, 191, 193, 195, 196, 197, 200, 204, 205, 207, 208, 209, 212, 213, 218, 221, 225, 229, 230, 231, 232, 233, 236, 237, 238
police, 125, 126, 130
policy, 11, 25, 36, 38, 46, 55, 57, 75, 81, 121, 131, 135, 136, 155, 161, 163, 167, 190, 193, 197, 199, 219, 226, 239, 247
policy issues, 167
policymakers, 17, 42, 192
population, 54, 77, 79, 112, 117, 119, 160, 168, 171, 181, 204, 209, 212, 224, 235, 248
population density, 117, 119, 160
poverty, xiii, 22, 54, 56, 71, 72, 94, 97, 109, 144, 152, 166, 175, 177
poverty line, 71
program administration, 91, 96, 116, 122, 128, 134, 137, 152, 155, 160, 225, 243
program outcomes, 237
programming, 124
project, 13, 17, 20, 56, 57, 74, 79, 100, 119, 120, 122, 127, 131, 133, 153, 162
proposed regulations, 6
public assistance, 185
public education, 95, 152
public health, 181, 196, 204
public policy, 204
public safety, 21

R

random assignment, 18
recommendations, 6, 24, 61, 62, 90, 100, 133, 137, 138, 153, 155, 162, 196, 197, 198, 199, 218, 219, 222, 239, 241, 248
regulations, xii, xiii, 5, 6, 9, 11, 12, 15, 16, 25, 26, 30, 36, 46, 50, 51, 61, 90, 94, 96, 98, 125, 139, 152, 154, 166, 169, 175, 179, 181, 182, 183, 185, 190, 192, 193, 197, 199, 204, 206, 207, 222, 223, 247
regulatory changes, 107, 158, 247
regulatory requirements, 99
reimburse, 73, 186, 237
reliability, 93, 94, 107, 137, 140, 141, 142, 159, 222, 236
requirements, ix, x, 2, 3, 5, 6, 7, 8, 9, 11, 12, 14, 15, 16, 18, 27, 28, 29, 30, 46, 61, 62, 63, 71, 73, 82, 97, 98, 99, 107, 108, 115, 125, 127, 128, 131, 134, 135, 136, 138, 146, 147, 152, 153, 158, 159, 161, 163, 173, 181, 188, 191, 192, 206, 207, 219, 220, 223, 224, 225, 226, 227, 228, 229, 230, 231, 232, 235, 240, 241, 245

resources, 13, 18, 22, 25, 47, 61, 62, 83, 112, 119, 124, 128, 185, 187, 193, 197, 220, 236, 237, 241, 243, 246, 247
response, 94, 107, 115, 129, 143, 146, 147, 160, 198, 221, 240, 243, 248
retail, xiv, 112, 166, 172, 184, 187, 189, 190, 192
revenue, 24, 26, 29, 30, 191, 192
risk, xiii, 37, 38, 49, 50, 69, 112, 134, 166, 167, 173, 178, 179, 180, 204, 207, 208, 220, 226, 246
rules, vii, viii, xiii, 2, 37, 38, 42, 49, 50, 53, 55, 57, 59, 62, 68, 71, 74, 111, 134, 166, 175, 183, 191, 197, 199, 223, 227, 245, 247
rural areas, 17, 20, 21, 100, 111, 116, 117, 119, 120, 147, 153, 160

S

safety, 92, 129, 130, 132, 133, 155, 160, 161, 162
school, vii, viii, ix, x, xi, xii, xiii, 1, 2, 3, 4, 5, 6, 7, 8, 9, 11, 12, 13, 14, 15, 16, 17, 21, 22, 23, 24, 25, 26, 27, 28, 29, 30, 31, 34, 36, 37, 38, 39, 40, 41, 42, 43, 44, 46, 47, 48, 49, 50, 51, 52, 53, 54, 55, 56, 57, 58, 59, 60, 61, 62, 63, 64, 65, 66, 67, 68, 69, 70, 71, 72, 73, 75, 76, 77, 78, 79, 80, 81, 82, 83, 84, 85, 86, 87, 88, 90, 91, 92, 95, 97, 98, 100, 101, 103, 106, 107, 108, 109, 110, 111, 112, 117, 120, 122, 123, 129, 133, 134, 135, 136, 142, 144, 147, 151, 152, 153, 156, 158, 159, 162,163, 165, 168, 175, 220, 224
School Breakfast Program, vii, viii, x, 1, 3, 5, 6, 9, 11, 14, 28, 31, 34, 39, 41, 43, 46, 49, 50, 59, 60, 61, 62, 65, 66, 69, 84, 89, 94, 141
school meals, v, vii, viii, ix, x, xiii, 1, 2, 5, 6, 7, 8, 9, 10, 11, 12, 14, 17, 21, 22, 23, 25, 26, 34, 36, 39, 46, 48, 50, 51, 52, 53, 55, 57, 58, 59, 60, 61, 65, 67, 68, 69, 71, 72, 75, 76, 77, 78, 80, 81, 82, 97, 111, 113, 117, 134, 139, 152, 163, 165, 168, 175
school meals programs, v, vii, viii, ix, x, 1, 2, 8, 12, 14, 17, 21, 25, 26, 36, 39, 46, 48, 50, 51, 52, 53, 55, 67, 168
Secretary of Agriculture, 12, 99, 132, 152, 162
self-employment, 225
self-sufficiency, 225, 233
Senate, 4, 12, 14, 16, 19, 21, 28, 30, 43, 99, 100, 132, 153, 162, 168, 187, 214
service provider, 99, 100, 152, 153, 236, 237
services, xiv, 34, 71, 73, 99, 100, 125, 126, 127, 133, 134, 153, 162, 166, 169, 170, 172, 178, 180, 184, 185, 187, 204, 218, 225, 232, 236, 237
SFSP participation, vii, xii, 90, 107, 123, 128, 140, 144, 154, 155, 158
social services, xii, 44, 97, 165, 167, 180, 208
social support, 71
sodium, viii, 2, 6, 7, 8, 9, 10, 11, 12, 61, 62
Special Milk Program, vii, viii, x, 1, 3, 5, 31, 34, 38, 39, 41, 43, 50, 69, 78, 84
Special Supplemental Nutrition Program for Women, Infants, and Children (WIC), vi, vii, viii, x, xii, 3, 17, 18, 33, 34, 35, 36, 37, 38, 41, 44, 57, 77, 79, 90, 109, 111, 112, 165, 166, 167, 168, 169, 170, 171, 172, 173, 174, 175, 176, 177, 178, 179, 180, 181, 182, 183, 184, 185, 186, 187, 188, 189, 190, 191, 192, 193, 194, 195, 196, 197, 198, 199, 200, 201, 203, 204, 205, 206, 207, 208, 209, 210, 211, 212, 213
spending, xi, 4, 35, 37, 40, 45, 48, 49, 68, 70, 81, 171, 191, 192, 193, 227

stakeholders, 5, 12, 106, 132, 137, 161, 186, 187, 222
strategic planning, 91, 106, 107, 136, 154, 157, 159
student enrollment, 57
subgroups, 209, 212, 228, 230, 231
subsidy, xi, 40, 42, 47, 54, 67, 72, 73, 83
Summer Food Service Program, vii, viii, x, 1, 3, 5, 16, 20, 31, 34, 39, 41, 43, 49, 69, 74, 77, 84, 87, 89, 91, 92, 93, 96, 102, 104, 110, 114, 116, 118, 124, 125, 126, 127, 138, 145, 146, 147, 148, 149, 150, 151, 156, 157
summer meals, v, vii, ix, xii, 2, 4, 16, 17, 65, 74, 75, 77, 89, 90, 91, 93, 98, 100, 108, 109, 110, 112, 113, 114, 115, 118, 119, 121, 122, 124, 130, 132, 133, 138, 141, 142, 143, 147, 151, 153, 154, 159, 160, 161, 163
summer program, 43, 44, 46, 81, 101
Supplemental Nutrition Assistance Program, vi, xiii, 17, 35, 42, 56, 89, 111, 112, 166, 173, 176, 218, 220, 222, 234, 241, 248

T

technical assistance, 6, 41, 61, 82, 83, 128, 143, 145, 169, 219, 238, 239, 241, 242
technical comments, 138, 213
time frame, 175, 176
time periods, 22, 125, 239
trafficking, xiv, xv, 218, 219, 220, 221, 227, 242, 244, 245, 246, 247, 248
training, 82, 83, 97, 191, 218, 220, 221, 224, 225, 226, 232, 236, 237, 238, 241, 243
training programs, 225, 236, 237, 238
transactions, 187, 191, 192, 227, 244
transportation, 117, 119, 160, 224, 227, 233, 237

U

U.S. Department of Agriculture Food and Nutrition Service (USDA-FNS), vii, viii, x, 1, 3, 5, 6, 7, 8, 9, 10, 11, 13, 15, 17, 18, 19, 20, 22, 24, 25, 26, 28, 30, 31, 38, 39, 42, 44, 46, 47, 50, 52, 55, 56, 59, 60, 61, 62, 63, 64, 66, 68, 70, 71, 74, 76, 77, 78, 79, 81, 82, 83, 84, 85, 86, 120, 122, 167, 168, 169, 170, 171, 174, 176, 178, 179, 181, 182, 184, 185, 186, 187, 190, 192, 193, 194, 196, 197, 198, 199, 200, 201

V

variations, 106, 137, 143, 159, 177, 195
varieties, 6, 191, 245
vegetables, vi, viii, ix, xiii, 2, 6, 7, 13, 15, 16, 18, 61, 70, 80, 98, 166, 181, 182, 191, 196, 197, 198, 199, 203, 204, 205, 206, 207, 208, 209, 210, 211, 212, 245
violence, 130, 132, 137, 161, 162
violent crime, 130, 161
vocational training, 232
vouchers, xiv, 34, 38, 166, 180, 184, 186, 199, 200, 205, 208

W

waiver, 15, 99, 100, 130, 131, 133, 152, 153, 161, 225, 235
WIC program, viii, 37, 167, 168, 169, 170, 171, 173, 174, 178, 180, 183, 187, 188, 189, 190, 192, 193
workforce, 226, 236, 237
workload, 115

Related Nova Publications

CHILDREN'S ISSUES AND LEGISLATION: SELECT ANALYSIS AND IMPLICATIONS

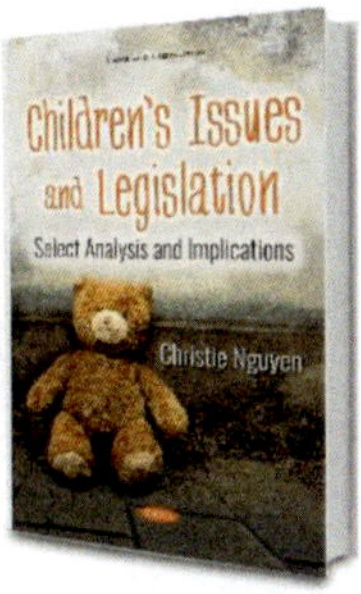

EDITOR: Christie Nguyen

SERIES: Laws and Legislation

BOOK DESCRIPTION: This book is a compilation of CRS reports on children's issues and legislation. Some topics discussed herein include runaway and homeless youth, unauthorized childhood arrivals, the Taxpayer Relief Act of 1997, the Missing Children's Assistance Act and the Deferred Action for Childhood Arrivals policy.

SOFTCOVER ISBN: 978-1-53614-493-2
RETAIL PRICE: $82

CHILDREN'S ISSUES AND CHALLENGES – CRS REPORTS FROM 2017 TO 2018

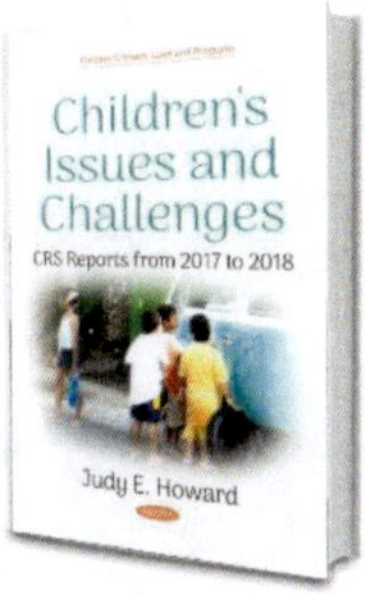

EDITOR: Judy E. Howard

SERIES: Children's Issues, Laws and Programs

BOOK DESCRIPTION: This book includes CRS reports from 2017 to 2018 and is focused on children's issues, such as unaccompanied alien children (UAC) runaway and homeless youth, the DACA Program as well as recent privacy and security issues associated with the increasing number of smart toys being created for children.

SOFTCOVER ISBN: 978-1-53613-822-1
RETAIL PRICE: $82

To see complete list of Nova publications, please visit our website at www.novapublishers.com